P9-EJU-718

The 90-Day Fitness
Walking Program

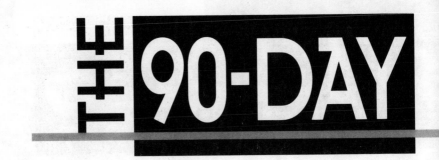

THE 90-DAY

FITNESS

WALKING
PROGRAM

Mark Fenton
and Seth Bauer,
editors of *Walking Magazine*®

A PERIGEE BOOK

A Perigee Book
Published by The Berkley Publishing Group
200 Madison Avenue
New York, NY 10016

Copyright © 1995 by Walking Magazine®

Book design by Irving Perkins Associates

Text illustrations by Walt Floyd

Cover design by Dale Fiorillo

First edition: April 1995

Published simultaneously in Canada.

Library of Congress Cataloging-in-Publication Data
Fenton, Mark.
    The 90-day fitness walking program / Mark Fenton and Seth Bauer.
        p.   cm.
    ISBN 0-399-51898-3
    1. Fitness walking.   2. Physical fitness.   I. Bauer, Seth.
    II. Title.   III. Title: Ninety-day fitness walking program.
    RA781.65.F46   1995
    613.7'176—dc20   94-32634
                                                          CIP

Printed in the United States of America.

10   9   8   7   6   5   4   3   2   1

This book is printed on acid-free paper.
∞

NOTICE: If you have never exercised before, are pregnant, are a man
over 40 or a woman over 50, or have a history of high blood pressure or
heart disease, it is recommended that you speak to your doctor before
beginning any exercise program, as a precautionary measure.

INTRODUCTION

Are you an athlete? No, you may say, I don't like sports—never have. Or maybe you *were* an athlete, but that was a long time ago. The fact is, we are all athletes. The human body is designed to *move.* Our anatomical systems—hearts, lungs, muscles, bones—were all meant to be part of an active being. If we stop moving, these systems begin to deteriorate—and they let us know it. We gain weight, lose muscle and bone, begin to have problems with our hearts. And if we stay sedentary for long enough, we increase the likelihood of receiving the ultimate sign of trouble: an early death.

The good news is that if you start moving and keep moving, these warning signs can disappear. The extra weight comes off, muscles and bones grow, hearts get stronger and signals of distress—high cholesterol and high blood pressure, among others—decrease in intensity. And research shows that this holds true no matter what age or sex or weight you are right now. It's never the wrong time to start.

This book, then, has a simple mission: It is meant to get you moving again. We believe that if people only knew how easy it is to gain the health benefits of walking, if they only understood the few simple principles behind a safe, effective exercise program, if they only realized how little extra effort it takes to fit walking into their days, no one would be sedentary. What will it take to create a totally active population? Education and motivation. Education, of course, is what *Walking Magazine* is all about. We want people to understand the hows and whys of exercise. The motivation comes from you—with our help.

You just took step one (no pun intended) when you bought this book. But don't expect to settle into a big armchair for a nice long read. This book is meant to be read in short segments, one each day for 90 days. If you're going to start a walking program, you want to spend your time walking, not reading.

Why walking? Aren't there a million other exercises that you could try? Isn't the ultimate goal to move, not necessarily to walk? Well, yes—and no. There are a host of reasons why walking is the most popular exercise in the United States. As we write this, polls show that more than 30 million Americans walk for exercise—14 million of them more than twice a week. There are 6 million more frequent walkers than frequent runners. And those 30 million walkers average 3 days each week and 2.92 miles per day. These statistics illustrate one reason to walk: Because walking is a low-impact activity, it's easy enough on your body that you can do it as often as you like—every day, if you choose. And walkers have a remarkably low number of activity-related injuries.

So that's the safety lesson. Here's another reason to walk: It's a fabulously effective fitness activity. There are all kinds of studies showing the clinical health benefits of walking, ranging from lowered blood pressure to reduced stress. But its effectiveness is proven to us much more vividly every day by the letters we receive from *Walking Magazine* readers. Their stories demonstrate that this simple activity can be positively life-changing. Like the story of one 23-year-old woman who weighed 260 pounds and felt shut out of society. A walking program led her to change her eating habits—and the combination of diet and exercise has taken off 112 pounds so far. Another reader felt that walking made her strong enough to leave an abusive marriage. And another said, "Walking is my Prozac." In short, there are many healthy and positive effects of walking.

Which leads us to the greatest reason to begin a walking program: the pleasure principle. Though this book contains a 90-day program, we obviously don't want you to walk for 90 days and then stop. The idea is to start moving now and to keep moving for the rest of your life. And let's face it: If you participate in an activity that you merely tolerate because you think it's good for you, you'll look for any excuse to stop. If you truly enjoy your exercise, though, you'll look for any excuse to participate. Pleasure makes walking a rest-of-your-lifetime activity. One which we hope you will enjoy as much as we do.

HOW TO USE THIS BOOK

The 90-Day Fitness Walking Program is designed to be your companion and advisor as you build a daily fitness walking habit. If you follow the program, by the end of the 90 days you will be walking 30 minutes per day, six days a week. This is the current recommendation for long-term health and well-being offered by the American College of Sports Medicine, the American Heart Association, and other health organizations.

Unlike most exercise books, you don't have to read this one all the way through before beginning your exercise program; nor do you have to run out and buy lots of gear or join a health club. Many would-be exercisers spend so much time and effort preparing to work out that they never actually get any exercise. This book is meant to answer your questions as they would typically arise during the normal course of beginning an exercise program, allowing you to focus on the most important thing: walking.

Each day, you read that day's topic (total reading time, about three minutes) and take your walk. By the end of the book your reading time will have taught you the basics of exercise physiology, walking for weight loss, walking technique, stretching and strengthening, and biomechanics. But you'll have taught yourself the critical lessons: how great walking can make you look and feel, and how to organize your day so that walking is a natural part of it. If you have three minutes to read Day One and 10 minutes to walk, you're ready to begin right now.

One note about the walking times that are suggested for each day: They are targeted for people who have been inactive for an extended period of time. No harm will come to more active people who simply follow the schedule to the letter, of course, but if you begin the program and find that you can comfortably do more, there is no reason not to. Use these descriptions to generally assess your current fitness level, and if you choose to, you can follow the recommendations:

Inactive: You have a job or lifestyle in which you spend very little time on your feet. You get no regular exercise. You tend to avoid activities like climbing stairs or walking uphill because they feel like a physical challenge.
Recommendation: Walk the amounts listed for each day.

Lightly Active: Your lifestyle often involves standing, carrying things, climbing stairs, or moving. You occasionally take part in recreational activities like walking or swimming, or do active housework like raking, mowing, shoveling, or vacuuming.
Recommendation: After the first week or two, add 5–10 minutes to each day's walk.

Active: Your lifestyle or job requires a good deal of movement and activity. You take part in recreational activities several times per month. You already walk once or twice a week.
Recommendation: Double the daily schedule. Your goal will be building up to one hour of walking six days a week.

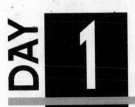

DAY 1 10 Minutes

Today you're going to begin a lifetime of fitness. Here's how: Walk out of your door and walk for five minutes in any direction at any speed. Then turn around and come home. That's it. You're done. You need no preparatory gyrations or incantations. You don't need to change clothes beforehand or shower afterward. Your workout is over.

Does that sound easy? It's supposed to. Does it sound like something that even the most out-of-shape person can handle? Exactly. So is it really a workout? It most certainly is.

Somehow, people have the notion that a workout is supposed to leave you tired and sore. We suspect that's precisely the reason why most Americans don't exercise: They try a "workout," they get tired and sore, and they quit. Or they simply imagine themselves getting tired and sore, and so they don't try to exercise in the first place.

In fact, for all but the most fit segment of society, a workout is any sustained exercise that you wouldn't have gotten in the normal course of your day. And if it doesn't leave you sore and tired, that's great. It means you're that much more likely to do tomorrow's workout—and the next day's. Everyone has heard that you're supposed to build up gradually, but few people who begin exercise programs actually build up gradually enough. That's why there are so many exercise drop-outs.

Another reason why 10 minutes is enough is that you're just in the first phase of your walking program. For a while,

FIVE MINUTES OUT, FIVE MINUTES BACK

the amount of exercise you get won't be nearly as important as simply building the habit. By the end of the 90 days, you will have moved (literally) through the three common phases: from habit-building, to increasing the depth of your exercise knowledge, to increasing the time and intensity of your walks.

So go take your 10-minute walk, and, to add to your sense of accomplishment (and perhaps to prove that it's a workout), make a check in the box at the bottom of this page.

5/5/15 = to Weber Cn Rd —
turn around + head home.

7-19-96   5:36 - 5:46pm

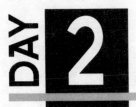

DAY 2
10 Minutes

Just like yesterday, find 10 minutes to walk. Note that we don't say "only" ten minutes, because a 10-minute walk is a very real first step to improving your health, fitness, and overall well-being. There is nothing "only" about the value of this walk. So make sure you find the time, whether first thing in the morning, during the day, just before or after dinner, or even late in the evening.

Whenever you fit it in, walk for ten minutes continuously. If a neighbor or coworker invites you to stop for a chat, either invite the chatterer to come along (it's perfectly fine to talk while you walk), or tell him or her you'll be back in about ten minutes, and would be happy to chat then.

Right now you are creating an important exercise habit, and you must convince yourself that this is valuable time, as important as anything you'll do for yourself during the day. Then you may have to convince others. So if that means you have to recruit family support, like asking a spouse to watch the kids, or—even better—getting them all to come along on their bikes, then do it. If it means mentioning to your boss that from now on you'll be walking at lunchtime, don't be worried. Remind them that walking is not only good for you, it will be good for those around you, as your fitness and energy levels rise, your attitude and self-image improve, and you just begin to feel better. Tell them that it may not happen overnight, but that it will happen, and you can use their help.

FIT IT IN AND CHECK IT OFF

As a basic safety measure, get in the habit of carrying an I.D., and 25¢ in case you need to make a telephone call. When you finish your walk, remember to check the box to indicate you did your ten minutes.

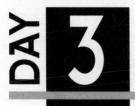

Once again, find ten minutes for a continuous walk. You may still simply head out your door, and walk five minutes out, then come back. Or, you may be developing a sense of about how far you walk in ten minutes, and so take a loop around the block. In any case, your goals on a 10-minute walk should be to have tall, healthy posture (no leaning forward from the waist, or slouching shoulders), and to move fairly continuously. A 30-second stop to wait for a light to change at an intersection is fine. A stop to discuss a neighbor's new hairdo or car is not. Similarly, if you take the dog along on your walk, a 5-second pause to sniff a tree is okay, but the elaborate 5-minute canine "meet and sniff" ritual with another neighborhood bowser is to be avoided.

There are both psychological and physical reasons to keep moving continuously. The psychological reason is that you're creating a new mindset, making your walk an important part of your day, worthy of a concentrated chunk of your time. The physiological reason is to make your heart pump a little harder for the full 10 minutes. Though some research indicates that exercise can be broken up into short bouts throughout the day without a significant reduction in benefits, 10 minutes is roughly what researchers have considered "short." Any less than that and it's unclear just what the physical effects will be.

Dress however you like on your walk—and wear the most comfortable pair of low-heeled shoes, athletic or other-

DRESS COMFORTABLY, AND DON'T STOP

wise, in your closet. You may find that padded athletic socks are more comfortable, but there are no rules. (Later, we'll discuss walking-specific clothing and shoes. For now, walking is much more important than buying. But if you feel discomfort in your feet or legs or start getting blisters, read Day 16.) You'll be fine with whatever clothes you've chosen for the day plus coats, hats and gloves as required by the season. The key is not to let the weather stop you. Unless the conditions are truly perilous—we're talking about lightning strikes or golfball-sized hail—you should be able to walk outdoors. Otherwise, find an indoor option: a treadmill, a local mall, or the halls at work.

Some people prefer to change their clothing specifically for their walk. They may have especially athletic or comfortable attire for walking, or they may just find that changing helps it feel more like a "real workout." You might try it to see if you like the ritual. But whatever you do, get in a 10-minute walk, and check it off below.

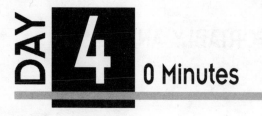

DAY 4 — 0 Minutes

Today is a day off from walking, or in sports parlance, *recovery*, which we'll discuss in tomorrow's entry, so you don't have to do a timed walk. However, that doesn't mean you shouldn't be thinking about fitness. In fact, now that you are becoming more active, one thing you can do to help your body is to drink plenty of water.

Things you may already know about water:

—Important in thermoregulation
—Key to maintenance of blood volume
—Helps you eliminate wastes
—Acts as an appetite suppressant
—Puts out fires

Water is a key to your body's temperature regulation system. As you heat up during exercise, your body sweats, and the evaporation of perspiration on your skin is an effective cooling process. The majority of your blood is water, so you must remain well hydrated for your body to maintain its full, healthy volume of blood. If your blood volume drops, it gets harder for your circulatory system to deliver oxygen and nutrients to the working muscles. Also, your kidneys need water as they work to clear your system of metabolic waste.

As you become more active throughout the day—and especially after your walk—you will probably be more thirsty. It's good to satisfy that thirst with water. But you

WHY YOU NEED WATER

should also drink water even when you don't feel thirsty. Your body is likely to need water whether you're thirsty or not.

Fortunately, not only does water fill your body's needs, but it also helps to fill your stomach. Drinking plenty of water (doctors recommend as many as eight 8-ounce glasses a day) can actually reduce your appetite somewhat, especially when you might otherwise be eating just for fun, rather than because you're hungry.

And yes, water does help with most fires (but remember, only use baking soda on those pesky kitchen flare-ups).

Since today is a day off, reward yourself for a healthy habit and check the box if you make a point of drinking an extra glass of water today.

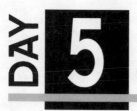

DAY 5 · 10 Minutes

Walk for ten minutes, continuously and purposefully. That means, walk as if you are trying to get somewhere. Walk as if it's a 10-minute walk to a store that closes in fifteen minutes, not as if you're sauntering to the car after an all-you-can-eat meal at a restaurant.

The reason you didn't walk yesterday is that you are introducing your body to something new, and it is important to give it recovery time—time to adjust to the workload. This relates to one of the fundamental characteristics of exercise—it elicits in your body a stress adaptation. You put your body under stress by asking it to do something it doesn't normally do, like walking for ten minutes. (Or, even if you walk ten minutes straight once in a while, you may not do it several days in a row, so that may be the stress.) In response to this stress, your body builds itself up a bit, trying to make itself capable of responding to the stress next time.

Because you're applying the load very gradually, with comfortable 10-minute walks, an occasional day off should be plenty to allow you to painlessly adapt. Still, you should monitor how you feel. Different bodies consider different things stressful. If you're overweight, or have really never exercised before, a purposeful 10-minute walk may stress your system. If you're already pretty active, then walking for ten minutes may not elicit much response from your body. In that case you may already find yourself very comfortable adding extra walking time. That's fine, and you can jot the

REST IS GOOD—JUST DON'T OVERDO IT

time you actually walk in the box, rather than simply checking it off. But in either case it's best to start very gradually, and to throw in a recovery day now and then to give your body tissues a chance to rebuild after the stress. We will discuss rebuilding later.

Now take your 10-minute walk (it's time for some stress—you rebuilt yesterday) and check it off.

TIME:

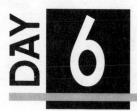

DAY 6
10 Minutes

This will be the last walk of your first week, so make sure you don't skip it. Since you're still in the first week, establishing the habit of getting out the door and walking whenever you wish is far more important than the distance or even the time involved.

Even with only one week of walking, you have begun to improve your health and well-being—especially your mental well-being. Though sometimes overlooked, the first positive effects of exercise tend to be psychological. Psychologists know that physical activity unleashes beta endorphin, the natural substance widely credited with causing "runner's high," and possibly other depression-reducing chemicals in the brain. They also feel that exercise may help the body reduce the level of stress-related hormones like cortisol. So, don't be surprised if you're feeling more relaxed and less tense after your walks. In fact, expect it.

If you are having trouble finding ten minutes a day for your walk, you should try formally scheduling one. We know people who write in the time for a daily walk in their personal calendars. Then they refuse to schedule anything else in that slot—it's as sacred as an appointment with the president! If that works for you, then do it. In fact, actually scheduling a walk can encourage others to join you.

"Nope, sorry Bob, 1:00 to 1:30 is no good. Got my walk scheduled in there. Of course, you're welcome to come along . . . if you think you can hack it." You can both

SCHEDULE IT, DO IT, AND CHECK IT

benefit from walking—and the buddy system can be a great motivator.

Start thinking about all the places you might like to take walks—the streets around home or work, a local park, a high school track, a nearby trail. In the long run, mixing up your routes will help you physically and mentally by varying the challenge and the view.

After your walk, remember to check the box. Two checks if you took Bob.

TIME:

DAY 7

0 Minutes

There is no walk scheduled for today (more rebuilding opportunity), but that doesn't mean you should turn into a slug. One way that you can continue to improve your health and fitness, even on days when you're not doing a formal, scheduled, timed walk, is to generally be more active. This is something you should be conscious of all of the time. A great deal of research examined by the American College of Sports Medicine and the National Centers for Disease Control establishes that simply being active in everyday life (taking the stairs instead of an elevator, walking a memo over to a coworker rather than sending it by interdepartmental mail, doing 15 minutes' worth of gardening or raking leaves) can have positive impacts on your health. That means a lower likelihood of cardiovascular disease and high blood pressure, and possibly greater longevity. When people go from simply being active to working regular exercise into their lives (say, a program of moderate-intensity walking), those benefits are greater: even lower rates of heart disease and hypertension, reduced chance of osteoporosis and colon cancer, less obesity, and even improved mental health.

You might be surprised by the number of calories consumed—a good indicator of how hard the work is—during everyday activities. In the chart, you can also see that heavier people tend to burn more calories, as they must move more body mass during activity.

STAY ACTIVE

Approximate calorie consumption for 15 minutes of the following activities:

Body Weight:	100 lbs	150 lbs	200 lbs
Dancing (ballroom):	35 cals.	53	69
Vacuuming:	44	66	88
Car washing:	48	72	93
Stacking firewood:	62	90	120
Lawn mowing:	78	114	152
Walking purposefully (about 3.5 mph):	59	92	117

Used by permission. From F. I. Katch and W. D. McArdle, *Introduction to Nutrition, Exercise, and Health,* 4th edition. Lea and Febiger, Philadelphia, 1993. Energy expenditure tables copyright © by Fitness Technologies, Inc., Amherst, MA.

What's the message? Look for ways to be more physically active all the time, not just when you're walking. For starters, do one more active thing today than you normally do (climb stairs, scrub the floor, play catch with your kids, wash the car) then check off the box below. And make it a habit to be more active. It does matter!

DAY 8

10 Minutes

For your 10-minute walk today, invite a friend. If you prefer to go alone, that's fine. But if you're married, or have a friend or a child who is curious about what you're up to, invite him or her along. Or grab a colleague at work who's been saying, "I should start working out," but never seems to get going. Why? Because it's good for you and good for the other person. Should your friend become a regular walking partner, you'll have an easier time continuing your program. As we said earlier, knowing that someone is depending on you to keep your walking date is great motivation.

But mostly you should invite someone simply because you enjoy his or her company, and you want that person to see how easy it is to accomplish a 10-minute walk, and how great you feel afterward. Because by now you are no doubt beginning to notice results. After your walk, you tend to be more alert and rejuvenated. That sense of being refreshed will strike whether it's a gorgeous spring day, or the middle of winter since your energy level is always higher after physical activity. One reason? Activity increases your heart rate and respiration, so more oxygen is coursing through your system and reaching your brain and nerve centers.

By the way, that's a hidden benefit of exercise that you can offer to your cohort. By raising your heart rate during a walk, not only do you burn more calories while you're active, but also during that period of elevated metabolism afterward. How many extra calories depends on your fit-

INVITE A FRIEND

ness level, and how long and how hard the exercise is. Longer and more intense exercise provides a greater calorie burn.

By now you may be venturing a bit farther on your walks. If so, you may occasionally run into a very territorial dog. If possible, cross to the other side of the street before reaching such an animal. But if an unleashed dog approaches you threateningly, short of sacrificing your walking partner you may find that the following advice helps: Don't run away, and do not act afraid. Face the dog, but make no threatening gestures. Speak in a firm, low but loud voice, and try, "Go home," "Stay," and even "Good dog." Walk away slowly, or back away if necessary. If it's a consistent problem, contact your local SPCA (Society for the Prevention of Cruelty to Animals) or police to notify them of the animal.

Check off the box after you walk for ten minutes, and write in the time if you go more than ten minutes.

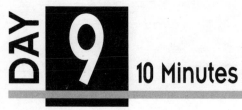

DAY 9 — 10 Minutes

You'll notice on the copyright page of this book, and on most written materials, tapes, or videos with an exercise prescription, a little warning not dissimilar to the one on those carnival signs which say if you're pregnant, or very overweight, or have a history of heart disease or a pacemaker, don't go on the "Spin 'til Your Eyes Pop Out" ride. For our purpose here, we add that if you're a man over 40 or a woman over 50, or if you've never engaged in exercise before, then you should consult your physician before beginning an exercise program.

Why is this important? All of the above groups are at a higher statistical risk than others of something like an irregular heartbeat or even a heart attack when they engage in moderate or vigorous exercise. (They apparently are also at higher risk when being spun 'til their eyes pop out.) So, it's a good idea to have your doctor check you out, and to make sure you understand the level of intensity at which you should be exercising. We have been going at a comfortable pace and for short time periods to this point,

CONSIDER A TALK WITH THE DOCTOR

so by and large you haven't been at risk. But if you do fall in one of those groups, it's important to call the doctor to discuss what you're doing, and to go in for a stress test if he or she thinks it is appropriate. More on that tomorrow.

Meanwhile, get in a 10-minute walk, and check it off.

_____

_____

_____

_____

_____

TIME: ☐

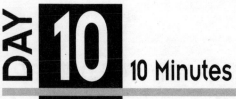

DAY 10

10 Minutes

Even if you're not in a high-risk group, you may want to see a doctor as you begin your exercise program to establish some physical benchmarks. By now, in your second week of walking, your body has already begun to change in some invisible ways. By learning some of your current measures of health, you can figure out over time just what your walking program does for you. And in the long run, that may be just the motivation you need to keep going.

Find out what your current weight, blood pressure, resting heart rate, total blood cholesterol, and HDL (that's high-density lipoprotein, the "good" cholesterol) levels are. Your doctor also may be able to measure your body fat percentage very simply with a pair of skin calipers, or at least discuss your current weight and waist-to-hip ratio with you. These numbers will give you some concrete data to

Health Measures:

	Around *Day 10*	Around *Day 85*	In 3–6 Months
Resting Heart Rate:			
Blood Pressure:			
Body Weight:			
% Body Fat:			
Total Cholesterol:			
HDL (good stuff):			
Other:			

HAVE THE DOCTOR CHECK YOUR CURRENT FITNESS LEVEL

compare in 10 or 12 weeks. Eighty days is an adequate amount of time to actually change some of those measurements, assuming you stay with your program.

It's also possible that the doctor will have you take a stress test. This test is actually an opportunity for doctors to watch how your body performs under progressive physical challenge. Typically, you are hooked up to heart-rate and blood-pressure monitoring equipment, and asked to walk on a treadmill. You begin slowly, and then move at higher speeds and up steeper inclines. Physicians watch for any irregularities in your heartbeat or blood pressure. If any are seen, they can then recommend thresholds or guidelines for physical activity (for example, no walking on extremely hot days, or never let your heart rate get above a certain level).

Walk for 10 minutes, and feel good that with each step you're making real progress toward improving all of those things you may have had monitored at the doctor's.

TIME:

DAY 11

0 Minutes

Today is a day off, but if for some reason you didn't do your walk for one of the last three days then take a 10-minute walk today and check it off below. Now you see one of the values of keeping a training log.

The simple activity of checking off a box, or writing how many minutes you have walked, has been creating a log of your activity. But not only is a log rewarding as you check it off, rightly congratulating yourself for that day's effort, it also creates a record of your walks. So now, if you don't recall exactly which days you walked, you can look back at the last three days and see whether they're all checked. If they are, then you can take today off.

If not, however, then walk ten minutes today. Your body has had plenty of rebuilding time lately, and it's ready for some more work. Otherwise, you won't be applying enough stress to keep improving your fitness level.

You may feel the program is starting slowly—that 10-minute walks will never get you in shape. But remember that this is the beginning of a very gradual buildup. At *Walking Magazine* we learn of hundreds of people each year that have huge successes based on modest beginnings. For example, Ron Cook began walking as an out-of-shape, 35-pound overweight 30-year-old, doing 5- and 10-minute strolls and covering far less than a mile. Within two years he had built enough endurance and conditioning to *walk* the 1994 Boston Marathon in just over 4½ hours, thus averaging about ten minutes per mile (6

CHECK YOUR TRAINING LOG

mph) for over 26 miles. So don't doubt your 10-minute walks. Just do them!

Last week we mentioned that you should be drinking plenty of water. This is a reminder that it should become a habit, on days you don't exercise as well as days you do. So drink two extra glasses of water over the course of the day, and check off below. (Or check off if you're making up for a missed walking day, and mark it as such.)

TIME:

DAY 12   10 Minutes

Why is it important not to miss your walks?

Because right now you are in the most critical phase of an exercise program: creating the habit. Over time we'll teach you how to walk farther and faster if you want, as well as how to make walking a total body exercise. But the most important thing we'll do is recommend six days per week of walking. And the most important thing you can do is to simply get in the habit of making the walk—even just ten minutes' worth—an absolutely central part of your day. It should be a part of your routine, as common as eating and brushing your teeth—but more fun.

Walking is such a healthy activity, you can do it six days a week without fear of injury. The impact force of your foot on the ground during a normal walking step is quite low, only about one to one and a half times your body weight (as opposed to three times body weight when running). And the movement is quite natural, so walkers suffer very few exercise-related injuries. Researchers at the University of Colorado compared the effectiveness of several exercise programs over a 28-week period, and found even ex-

DON'T TAKE EXTRA DAYS OFF

tremely fast fitness walkers averaged about 1.5 days missed because of injury, while runners missed more than 11 days. Yet, both groups enjoyed the same fitness benefits.

Remember to check the box after your 10-minute walk today.

TIME:

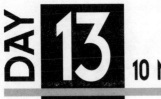

DAY 13 10 Minutes

You're probably finding that sometimes your walk is a minute or two longer than ten minutes, sometimes a minute shorter. As long as you don't make a habit of coming up short, this isn't a problem. Or, you may find you're regularly walking a few minutes longer. If you're feeling comfortable and doing that with ease, then don't stop. In fact, you should give yourself credit for the amount of time you've walked, so begin writing that time in the box, rather than simply checking the box. Even if you're following this program to the minute, you can write in the time. In the next few days you're going to begin increasing the length of your walks, and your log may be more helpful to you if you specifically write down how long they take.

You'll also notice that there is a line above the box labeled "where." That's so that you can record where you walked. Your entry can be as simple as "Flatus Park," or as detailed as "to the post office on 1st St., via Elm, and back." You may find you'll develop codes, like "the firehouse course," without listing the four streets that make up the loop. Recording this, combined with the actual time it took to do your walk, will let you do two things. You can watch your fitness improve over time (a route that now takes 12 minutes may take only 10 or 11 in a few weeks), and you can construct longer routes by putting shorter ones together (make a 20-minute walk by joining two 10-minute walks).

So, take a 10-minute walk today, and write in the

WRITE IN YOUR ACTUAL
WALKING TIME

time (whether it's 10, 9, or 14 minutes), and where you went for your walk. If logging the specifics isn't important to you, then just walk and check it off.

WHERE:

TIME:

Different people have different styles for making a walk a part of their day. Some people create firm plans, and let everyone around them know the importance of the walk. "I'll be leaving at two-thirty this afternoon, at which time I will drive to the park, to take my walk," they might announce, making clear that no one is to schedule anything during this now-sacred time. Others may simply slip out the door without a plan, because they feel like walking at that particular moment. Some people go through elaborate preparations, changing into specific walking attire and footwear; while others head out in whatever they have on.

There is no correct, universal style of walking. You must simply do what is most comfortable for you. And you may find it helps if it's comfortable for those around you. Some people are early-morning walkers—they get up 30 minutes before anyone else in the house, enjoy the absolute solitude of an early-morning walk, and are energized and ready to start the day when everyone else arises and it's time to begin chores, pack lunches, get ready for work, or take children to day care. Some couples find their daily walk is the only guaranteed time they have together, so it is planned and counted on for the 20 minutes after dinner each evening. In those cases, and millions of other routines, the schedule works well for everyone, and thus is easy to maintain.

Your walking style should include an eye toward safety. If

DEVELOP YOUR OWN "STYLE" FOR FINDING TIME TO WALK

you walk on roads, always walk facing the traffic. If you're walking in the dark, don very bright clothing, or even better, a reflective vest or shiny tape on your regular walking attire (most athletic stores have such gear). The best thing you can do is carry a small flashlight. Though it may not add much to your vision, it will make you vastly more visible to cars. And don't wait for total darkness to worry about visibility—the gray light of dawn and dusk can be equally dangerous.

Find your best time, take a 10-minute walk, and record where you went and how long you walked below.

WHERE:

TIME:

DAY 15 10 Minutes

Although walkers suffer very few injuries due to their exercise, one of the problems that does occasionally crop up is shin soreness. Some people call them shin splints, although that is an overused and very general term for a wide range of ailments of the lower leg. For walkers, especially novices, it is usually attributable to suddenly asking muscles on the front of your shin (the tibialis anterior) to do more work than they are prepared for. This is because on each walking step you land on your heel, and your shin muscles work to hold the toes up as they slowly roll to the ground. In fact, if your shins get sore enough, you may actually feel your foot flop down and hear your toes slap the ground during each step.

One way to help the shin muscles is to prepare them before your walk by warming them up slightly. An easy set of ankle circles will help get blood and oxygen flowing to these infrequently used fibers, and make the tissue warmer and more compliant. Simply stand on one foot, and, while holding the other off the ground, make circles in the air with your toes (you may need to hold onto something or someone for balance). Hold the leg steady, so that the circle comes just from rolling the ankle. Do five to ten in each direction, slowly, and make the toe circles as large as possible by moving the ankle through its full range of motion, then repeat for the other foot.

Do these before your walk, and stop in the middle for a few if you need to loosen up a tight shin. Another way to

DO ANKLE CIRCLES AND TOE POINTS FOR YOUR SHINS

stretch the shin is to simply lift the foot, point the toe, and hold it for a count of ten. These toe points are also a nice easy stretch for after your walk (even while sitting with a glass of water, for example).

Between ankle circles and toe points, get in a nice 10-minute walk, and record it below.

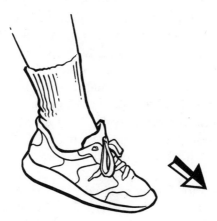

WHERE:

TIME:

DAY 16

0 Minutes

Today is a day off from walking, but an ideal day to do an equipment assessment. Another possible culprit in shin soreness is poor footwear, so here are the basic features of a sound shoe for walking.

If the heel of the shoe you're wearing while walking is very thick (either a dress shoe that is really built up and stiff, or even a thick-heeled athletic shoe), it may act as a lever as your heel strikes the ground, pulling the toes down too quickly and yanking on the shin muscle. So one feature of an ideal walking shoe is a slightly lower heel, especially as compared to built-up running shoes. The heel of a good walking shoe will also have a slight bevel or be rounded off (see sketch) to accommodate the heel strike.

You will also benefit if your shoes are flexible near the ball of the foot. That is where your foot naturally flexes as you push off with each step, so the shoe should flex there, too.

A walking shoe does not need to provide a great deal of lateral (side-to-side) support, since walking is a very straight-ahead motion. Thus, a high-top design (like some basketball and aerobics shoes) or support straps and layers may be overkill, adding unnecessary weight and heat retention to the shoe.

Finally, your shoe should fit properly. This means there should be a thumbnail's width of space between your toe and the end of the shoe when standing (your toes should never hit the end); your heel should not slip in and out

PICK COMFORTABLE FOOTWEAR

during a step; and there should be no friction points between your foot and the shoe. A large number of people wear shoes that simply don't fit very well—and then they're surprised when they have sore feet or blisters. So, give your shoes the once-over, and find the ones in the closet that best fit the bill. Or if none do, consider a purchase. You're a serious walker, and you deserve the best.

Check off if you do six ankle circles on each foot today, even if you've just done them while you were sitting and reading this.

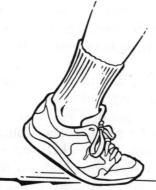

WHERE:

DAY 17
15 Minutes

Today you begin the important process of gradually increasing the amount of time that you walk. To allow your body to keep up with the changes, you will do this in very small increments, never increasing the walk on a given day by more than five minutes over the previous day, and never increasing the total time you walk in a week by more than about 10 to 20 percent.

So today, rather than walking out five minutes and coming back, you should walk 7½ minutes before turning around. You've now been walking long enough that this won't seem at all taxing. You may already be occasionally walking for fifteen minutes or more, which is fine—but don't feel any urgency to exceed our recommendations, or to get ahead of the program.

On the other hand, it may be difficult for you to find ten minutes in the day, and finding five more could seem impossible. That's another reason for the increases in walking time to be gradual. Your job is to continue to evolve your walking style to keep up with your walking schedule, and to keep your body on its schedule of improving fitness and health. So if that means the alarm clock is set five minutes earlier in the morning (and the

TAKE IT UP A NOTCH—OUT 7½ MINUTES, AND BACK

TV is shut off five minutes earlier the night before), make the commitment and do it. Your walk should be that important to you.

Take a 15-minute walk, and record the time and possibly the new course below.

_____

_____

_____

WHERE:

_____

_____

_____

DAY 18
10 Minutes

You'll notice that we drop back to a 10-minute walk today, and go back up to 15 again before the week is out. That's because our bodies appreciate that kind of variation in an exercise program. Rather than simply adding two minutes per day to every walk, you'll add five minutes to some days, and leave the other days at 10-minute walks. That allows you to stress the body a bit more on the 15-minute walks. But because you're so accustomed to walking ten minutes now, your body will actually be able to do some of its rebuilding on those days. This is really just a simplified version of a basic hard-easy training principle that coaches use with competitive athletes—follow hard training days with easier days to allow some recovery.

Now, admittedly, when we're talking about 10- and 15-minute walks, it may not seem the stress is great enough to make that much difference. But it depends entirely on how fit you were when you started this program. And more importantly, it's best to develop good habits, so that as you walk farther and faster, you know how to safely vary the exercise stress you place on your body. And the principle of

VARIETY IS A GOOD THING—AND OUR BODIES APPRECIATE IT

alternating harder and easier days may be valuable as you unleash the athlete within you, however fast or far you eventually choose to walk.

For now, enjoy a 10-minute "easy day," and record the details.

WHERE:

TIME:

Statements such as "lose 10 pounds in 10 days" have raised our expectations for rapid weight loss, without any thought for safety and health. Fortunately, a great many nutritionists and exercise physiologists have examined the question of weight loss very closely, and one verdict is absolutely crystal clear: The most effective and long-lasting weight loss and weight maintenance "programs" are simply based on combining a healthy, intelligent diet, with regular, moderate exercise.

A combination of diet and exercise may lead to losing as little as one to two pounds every two weeks. But that is a safe and healthy rate of weight loss, and once you create good habits, that rate can be maintained for as long as it

Estimated Calories Burned in 15 Minutes of Walking

Body Weight:	*100 lbs*	*150 lbs*	*200 lbs*
2.0 mph:	35 cals.	54	72
2.5 mph:	44	66	88
3.0 mph:	53	75	102
3.5 mph:	59	92	117
4.0 mph:	68	99	132

Used by permission. From F. I. Katch and W. D. McArdle, *Introduction to Nutrition, Exercise, and Health*, 4th edition. Lea and Febiger, Philadelphia, 1993. Energy expenditure tables copyright © by Fitness Technologies, Inc., Amherst, MA.

WHEN DO I START LOSING WEIGHT?

takes you to reach your ideal weight! Of course, the diet is best if it's normal food (not miracle potions or supplements in pill form), because you're most likely to stick with normal food for a lifetime. Your exercise should be enjoyable and easy to maintain, too, for the same reason. That's why walking is the perfect choice.

The bottom line in losing weight, say the experts, is your calorie balance: how many calories you take in during the day, compared to how many calories your body burns. This is the most important factor in determining your weight. For the most part, if you eat more than you burn over an extended period, you'll gain weight; burn more than you eat, and you'll lose weight. Note on the chart the faster you walk, and more body mass you carry, the more calories your walking will burn.

More details on diet, exercise, and weight over the next few days. Today, walk ten minutes (and burn some calories), then record your effort.

_____

_____

WHERE:

_____

_____

TIME:

DAY 20 — 15 Minutes

One reason we hear so much about cutting fat out of our diets and burning fat out of our bodies is that when we have an excessive intake of calories, our bodies store many of those calories as fat. Another reason is that dietary fat is high in calories (one gram of fat provides 9 calories, while a gram of carbohydrate has about 3.5 calories). And, since fat is often found in foods that are not as nutritious as foods with lots of carbohydrates it is often the culprit we are encouraged to reduce. But for weight loss, what you really should focus on is *balancing the calories you take in with the calories you burn.*

The best way to reach that calorie balance is not with strict calorie counting and hourly weigh-ins, but with a healthy combination of diet and exercise. (However, if you're numerically neurotic, on Day 50 we'll show you how to roughly estimate your daily caloric needs.) Either a diet or exercise alone *can* elicit changes in body weight, but neither is as effective—or as healthy—by itself.

For example, if you simply reduce your calorie intake you can lose some weight even without exercise. But it won't be the type or amount of weight that you ultimately want to lose, and it won't necessarily stay lost. Some of that weight you lose by dieting alone can be your lean body mass, or muscle—the best calorie-burner your body has! Having less muscle mass will in turn decrease your body's daily calorie requirement, so that to continue to lose weight, you must consume fewer and fewer calories. Other-

WHY DIET ALONE ISN'T THE ANSWER

wise, your body can plateau at the new weight. You can even begin to gain weight back—much of it fat, if you're not building muscle with exercise! Though this is a simplification of some complex physiological processes, it does help explain the yo-yo weight losses and gains that pure dieters often experience.

All the more reason to get out for fifteen minutes of walking exercise today, and log it.

WHERE:

TIME:

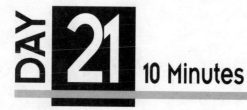

DAY 21 · 10 Minutes

Just as dieting alone may allow only limited weight loss, exercising alone without moderating your calorie intake is also a problem. A person can only burn so many calories in a single daily workout. And exercise generally tends to build muscle. So if you have only a small weekly caloric deficit (burn more than you eat) through exercise, you may replace some of the lost fat with muscle, and your net weight loss will be disproportionately small. The good news is that any muscle you create gives you more calorie-burning tissue, so you are heading in the right direction. But consider some hypothetical numbers:

Walking burns calories at different rates, depending on factors such as how fast you walk, how much you weigh, the terrain, and your fitness level (see Day 19 for some typical numbers). But a fairly fit, 150-pound person walking at a comfortable but purposeful 3-mph pace will burn about 300 calories in an hour of walking. Yet, one pound of body fat is equivalent to about 3500 calories. That's a lot of 15-minute walks! (By the way, other forms of moderate exercise don't burn any more.) Clearly, our 150-pound person

EXERCISE BY ITSELF WON'T KEEP WEIGHT OFF

needs to moderate her calorie intake, too, if weight loss is a goal.

Before you give up walking, crying that the road to weight loss is paved with misleading 90-day exercise programs, get out and take a 10-minute walk, and come back tomorrow—there are more factors to consider.

WHERE:

TIME:

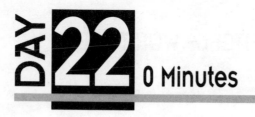

There are reasons why you should only expect to lose one to two pounds every two weeks, and by now you should be beginning to see why. Two days ago we saw that just dieting doesn't appear to be the answer to maintaining a healthy weight, as that can cause you to lose muscle as well as fat. Yesterday we saw that moderate exercise alone, especially when you're in the early stages of walking and just building up stamina, doesn't burn an extraordinary number of calories. But yesterday's was a worst-case analysis, and you will have many more factors working for you.

First, we're not stopping at 15-minute walks—this is only a part of our gradual buildup. Just doubling our daily jaunts to 30 minutes each would cut in half the time needed to lose a pound.

Second, if you weigh more than average or are less physically fit, you actually burn more calories walking at the same speed as a thinner person because you have to work harder. So the unfit shouldn't despair.

Third, as your fitness improves you'll naturally tend to walk faster, which also increases calorie consumption.

Fourth, there's that hidden benefit of the slight increase in your metabolism after your walk. How high the increase depends on how hard you've worked, but you'll certainly keep burning calories at an increased rate for some time after you've completed your walk.

And finally, as you begin to build those walking muscles, they will actually continue to burn more calories *all* the

WHY EXERCISE IS THE KEY TO WEIGHT MAINTENANCE

time. This means that even your "resting" metabolism—
that sitting-around-reading-a-book calorie consumption—
goes up as you build muscle and improve in fitness. All of
these factors improve the weight-loss benefits of exercise.
And though they are not instantaneous, they are lasting
changes as long as you stick with a walking program.

Perhaps the most important benefits, however, occur
when you also improve your diet. More on that tomorrow.
For today, remind yourself that one of the first important
steps to a healthier diet is drinking plenty of water (but, of
course, you already know that), and check off below if you
drink an extra glass of water today.

WHERE: _____

DAY 23

10 Minutes

The last piece of the diet-and-exercise puzzle that's important to know, whether you're trying to lose weight or not, is that the very foods that are better for weight loss are also better fuel for an exercising body. So all of the basic advice that's given to a dieter—cut back on fat, eat more fresh fruits and vegetables, whole grains, and legumes, and drink lots of water—is also perfect advice for the budding walker. (You only have to look at the Department of Agriculture's Food Guide Pyramid for those suggestions.)

Your muscles are looking for fuel to burn when you go out and walk each day, and the easiest foods to convert into muscle fuel are complex carbohydrates. That's the sugar in most fruits and vegetables, and the starch in many whole grains and legumes. Plus, the fibers in fruits, vegetables, and whole grains are thought to have other positive effects, from aiding in digestion to reducing the risks of some types of cancer. So don't make food choices lightly—really think about what you're eating.

As a first step, try to think of ways to replace fatty foods with low- or non-fat options that you can still enjoy. Consider jam on a bagel instead of cream cheese. Try mustard instead of mayonnaise on a sandwich, and have a piece of fruit after lunch rather than a cookie. Start with your next meal.

Now take a 10-minute walk, and make your muscles consume some fuel.

A HEALTHIER DIET WILL HELP YOUR FITNESS WALKING, TOO

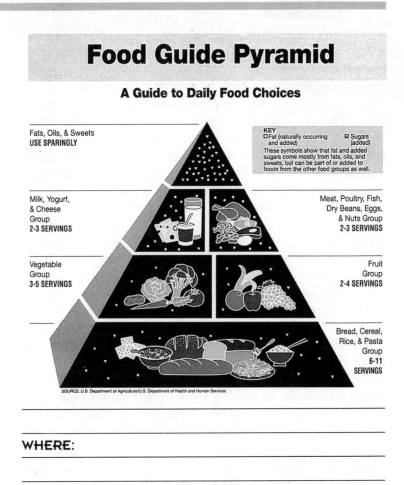

Food Guide Pyramid

A Guide to Daily Food Choices

Fats, Oils, & Sweets
USE SPARINGLY

KEY
☐ Fat (naturally occurring and added) ☑ Sugars (added)
These symbols show that fat and added sugars come mostly from fats, oils, and sweets, but can be part of or added to foods from the other food groups as well.

Milk, Yogurt, & Cheese Group
2-3 SERVINGS

Meat, Poultry, Fish, Dry Beans, Eggs, & Nuts Group
2-3 SERVINGS

Vegetable Group
3-5 SERVINGS

Fruit Group
2-4 SERVINGS

Bread, Cereal, Rice, & Pasta Group
6-11 SERVINGS

SOURCE: U.S. Department of Agriculture/U.S. Department of Health and Human Services

WHERE:

TIME:

DAY 24

15 Minutes

You've been walking for three weeks now, and we haven't once mentioned trying to measure the speed you're walking. You've simply walked at a purposeful, you-are-trying-to-get-somewhere, but comfortable, not-so-fast-that-it-hurts pace. The reason we don't focus on speed is that right now you're creating basic, lifelong habits, not necessarily trying to walk faster or farther. The first, and most important, habit to develop is getting out to walk regularly. Every day you stick with the program and log your minutes, you strengthen that habit.

The second habit is to introduce changes to your body gradually. So, you add five minutes to your walk every once in a while, but you don't pile on the minutes all at once. You also follow the hard-easy principle, varying your distances within a week.

The third habit is to combine your exercise with a healthy diet. Every time you trade a fatty food for something healthy, or drink some water rather than eat a snack you don't need, you work on that habit.

Now it's time to add an additional habit: maintaining a healthy and natural walking technique. First and foremost is a tall, upright posture. We all know people who are five feet, four inches tall, but appear much taller because of how they carry themselves. And we know people who are six feet, three inches tall, yet seem downright diminutive or gawky because they always slouch and look at the ground. They don't walk tall, they walk frumpy.

TO WALK "RIGHT," WALK NATURALLY

On your 15-minute walk today, don't be a frump. Walk as tall as your genetics will allow.

WHERE:

TIME:

DAY 25
10 Minutes

The rules for good walking posture are the same rules for posture your mom used to give you:

Don't stare at the ground—keep your head up and your eyes forward. Don't slouch. But don't scrunch your shoulders up to your ears—keep them relaxed. Be tall. And no shelf-butt.

Okay, maybe she didn't say no shelf-butt, but she should have. That's because it's unhealthy to arch your lower back and let your rear stick out. Doing this can lead to lower back soreness. To avoid shelf-butt (often called sway-back), very gently contract your abdominal muscles while walking to help pull in your stomach and flatten your lower back.

None of this is unnatural, and none of this should feel forced—it's all part of good, healthy posture. So, you should think about these things all the time, not just when you're walking.

Today you have a short 10-minute walk scheduled, so concentrate on tall posture throughout. And do a few ankle circles beforehand to warm up and strengthen your shins.

WALK TALL: HEAD UP, SHOULDERS RELAXED, AND NO SHELF-BUTT

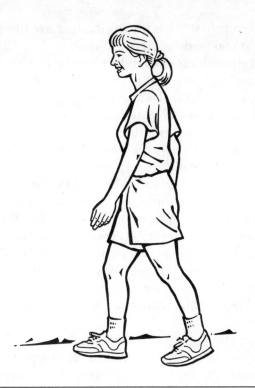

WHERE:

TIME:

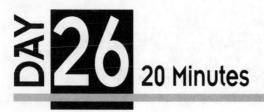

DAY 26 20 Minutes

Today is your first 20-minute walk. Just five minutes more than what you've done up until now, and you'll no doubt find there's nothing to it. In fact, maybe you're already out there sneaking 20-minute walks. Or, check your log—perhaps some of your 15-minute walks came in at 17 or 18 minutes. The point is, you'll have no problem physically walking for 20 minutes. (If you can walk 10 to 15 minutes without stopping at a purposeful pace practically every day of the week, you can certainly walk 20.)

Once again, the issue may be finding the time for a 20-minute walk. Ten minutes wasn't much, but now we're up to a whole third of an hour of your busy day. This is where you have to hang tough! You're already beginning to feel the value of your walks—increased energy, sleeping better at night, a bit of weight loss, even a better self-image. Well, have confidence that those benefits and more will continue as long as you continue to make your walk important enough to do every day!

As you're beginning to walk longer, you should make the first few minutes of your walk a warm-up. That simply means start your walk very slowly and comfortably—at a stroll, rather than your eventual purposeful pace. Just three to five minutes of very easy strolling allows your body to come up to exercise temperature very gradually (hence the term "warm-up"). Warmer muscles are less prone to injury or next-day stiffness, and your body opens the oxygen throttle from your lung's airways to the capillaries

START WITH EASY STROLLING

(tiny blood vessels) carrying oxygen to the muscles. And though you're not working at such a high intensity that it's critical right now, as you get more fit, your purposeful walking pace will get faster, and the benefits of a few minutes of easy warm-up will be greater.

Start with easy strolling and then continue on for a total walk of 20 minutes (warm-up included). Record the time and course of your walk.

WHERE:

TIME:

DAY 27
10 Minutes

As part of your healthy walking technique, you should be using your natural stride length. Some people try to really reach out with their heel and take as long a stride as possible when walking purposefully, but that's unnecessary. In fact, biomechanical research shows that the faster we walk, the more we depend on *quickening* our steps rather than *lengthening* them. (That's logical, because there are physical limits to how long a stride a person can take; namely, the length of his legs.) So, when you speed up from your warm-up pace to your purposeful pace, don't try to reach for a longer stride—it will come by itself. Instead, concentrate on taking quicker steps.

To see if you're pretty close to a natural step length, try the following exercise: Stand on an imaginary line with both feet together. Slowly lean forward from the ankles, keeping your body straight. That is, don't bend forward at the waist, just from your feet, until you begin to feel like you're falling. Then step forward as naturally as you can to catch yourself. That step is a fairly natural length for you, and no longer. This is a good exercise because walking is really a series of very tiny falls forward, in which we catch ourselves on our forward foot, then lift the opposite leg and fall into the next step.

Don't overstride by reaching for the next step—simply fall into it on your 10-minute walk today.

FALL INTO YOUR NATURAL STEP

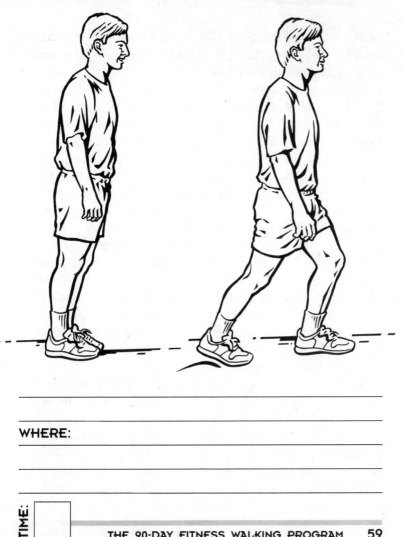

DAY 28 15 Minutes

After today's 15-minute walk, you will have completed four weeks of serious walking. Depending on your fitness level when you started, your body is probably already responding to your new activity level. For example, the volume of blood coursing through your arteries is one of the first things to respond to exercise. So believe it or not, you're likely to have more blood in your body than you did last month. And that's making delivery of oxygen to your muscles more efficient. This is only one of the subtle changes your body will go through as you get in better shape.

Tomorrow is scheduled as a day off, followed by six continuous days of walking (as you've done this past six days). By now, you've probably already determined what kind of schedule works for you. But if you're still having questions about what part of the day works best, try adding a bit of information to your training log. Jot down the time of day you walk next to "when" (something simple, like "6 am" or "lunchtime"), and record how your walk went, next to "how." Just write how you felt, whether you enjoyed it, whatever strikes you.

After several weeks of logging this, you may notice a pattern. If all your early-morning walks have comments like "felt sluggish" and "no fun—not awake yet," or a subtle "hated it!" then maybe that's not your best time of day to walk. But if you have comments like "felt great—lots of zing in my legs" or "gorgeous morning," while your afternoon walks say "body felt beat," you may decide to

RECORD THE TIME OF DAY, AND HOW YOU FEEL

walk in the morning, when your energy and optimism are highest.

You will also notice other factors that influence your walks by keeping this log. For example, if lunchtime walks at work always end up being shorter than you intend, it may mean you're feeling time pressure, and you should see if you can adjust your schedule, or walk before or after work instead. If your comments reflect exhaustion on a certain hilly course through the neighborhood, save that loop for your more energetic days.

Go out and walk 15 minutes whenever you choose, then try logging your comments in a permanent record.

WHEN: _____ AM/PM

HOW: _____

WHERE: _____

_____

_____

TIME: ☐

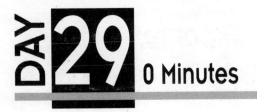

DAY 29 0 Minutes

Today is a day off, but you'll walk for six days before your next day off. This schedule will be the pattern for the rest of the 90-day program—six days on and one day off. That's because your ultimate goal for long-term health should be, according to the American College of Sports Medicine's 1993 guidelines, to get in regular, moderate-intensity activity, most days of the week.

This is one of the most important reasons why you keep a training log. Sure, it's great to record the loops that you walk, and see how you cover more distance in the same time as you get in better shape. And certainly it's valuable to watch for patterns in your walking routine, to determine the best times to walk, and even best people to walk with (you may notice you always get a nice vigorous workout with one cohort, but never seem to get that with another chatterbox). But the single most important thing your log will let you do is make sure you're walking most days of the week. You can simply look back when you reach a scheduled day off (today, for example), and if you've missed a day in the preceding week make up for it by taking a short 10-minute walk on the day off—today.

You may also choose to look ahead to the next six days and adjust your walking times based on your schedule if necessary. So, if you're going to be really busy on Day 32, just do a 10-minute walk that day, and take the scheduled 20-minute walk on Day 31 instead. Just be sure to follow the hard-easy principle, so if you're finding 20-minute walks

WALK MOST DAYS OF THE WEEK

a little more challenging, keep them spread out over the week rather than bunched together. And try to make the total number of minutes you walk still total the goal for seven days.

Enjoy a day off (it's okay to write "0" in the box), unless you missed one last week. If so, walk 10 minutes today and log it.

WHEN: AM/PM

HOW:

WHERE:

TIME:

DAY 30 15 Minutes

Are you still thinking about a tall walking posture and a natural, quick step? This is an image you should ingrain, because it is the basis for a lifetime of healthy walking. Everything else you may hear about walking technique, like pushing off with your back foot to generate more power, or bending your arms for speed, may be true. But the basics you never want to forget are a tall, relaxed posture and a quick, easy stride.

Here's a simple drill to use as a posture check: Stand with your back to a wall about a foot away from it, with your feet spread shoulder-width apart, and your knees slightly bent. Lean against the wall, with your back, head, shoulders, and rear touching it. Then slide one hand between the small of your back and the wall, to see how much of an arch you naturally have there. This arch creates the infamous shelf-butt (Day 25). Now, gently contract your abdominal muscles. Tighten them so you feel like you're pulling your pelvis slightly up toward your chest. Feel how the small of your back pulls in toward the wall? This is how gently contracting your abdominal muscles helps to protect your lower back—by reducing that arch.

If you don't feel much of an arch in this position, stand with your heels up against the wall (keeping your head, shoulders, and rear against the wall, too) and see if you can still tighten the abdominals and bring the small of the back into the wall.

To turn this into a little exercise to help your walk,

UP AGAINST THE WALL—TO CHECK YOUR POSTURE

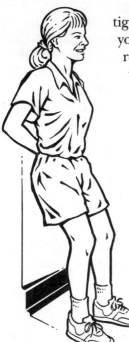

tighten your abdominals to flatten your back and count slowly to ten, then relax for five seconds. Repeat that three more times. This is an ideal exercise to do as a warm-up, combined with your ankle circles (remember Day 15?) for about two minutes before your walk.

Do a set of these posture checks, and some ankle circles (just to remind yourself) before your 15-minute walk today.

WHEN: _____ AM/PM

HOW: _____

WHERE: _____

_____

_____

TIME: ☐

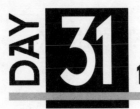

DAY 31
10 Minutes

Notice that you're continuing to slowly add minutes to your walks. This is to keep very gently stressing the body, so that it responds by making you a better walking machine. As we continue to throw in very easy days (like today's 10-minute walk) to give you a physical break and make the change gradual, you'll notice that the total number of minutes you walk in a week still never increases more than about 20 percent from one week to the next. This may not seem critical when we're dealing with 10-to-20-minute walks, and you may even be saying, "Oh, come on, this isn't even hard. I feel fine." Well, *that's the idea!* You're supposed to feel fine—that's what keeps you coming back and walking tomorrow. If you were waking up each day thinking, "Man, am I tired and sore. I'm not even opening up that stupid book today!" then we'd have a problem. So, keep feeling fine, and keep walking.

Which doesn't mean you should be bored. If you've consistently been doing a bit more than the recommended amount of walking and need that challenge to stay interested, and if your walks are enjoyable and you're feeling healthy and well rested doing so, then keep it up. Simply try to follow the pattern laid out here, varying your walks from day to day, and log your walking time accurately so you can keep an eye on the total number of minutes you walk each week. Then, you can accurately monitor your walking so you don't make a 50 percent increase in total minutes all in one week.

BUILDING UP YOUR WALKS

The other reason the change is gradual is to help you to keep incorporating walking into your life. More on that tomorrow. Today, walk 10 minutes (or more if you're inclined) and record the details.

WHEN: _____ AM/PM

HOW: _____

WHERE: _____

_____

_____

TIME: [ ]

DAY 32 20 Minutes

The habit of daily walking may really be feeling quite normal to you—you've been doing it for a month, after all. But the other reason you increase your walking time gradually (besides allowing for physical adaptations and rebuilding) is so that you keep making your walks an integral part of the day. As they begin to demand more time (20 minutes now instead of 10, and in another few weeks 25) you've got to figure out how to make your walks fun, and fit right into your lifestyle—important enough never to be missed, and fun enough so that you look forward to them.

Some suggestions:

Explore new places. Twenty minutes is long enough to actually get somewhere, so walk somewhere you enjoy or would like to explore such as a part of town you like, or a park you drive by but rarely visit.

Walk for errands. Find out if twenty minutes is long enough for a round trip to the post office, or to the store where you pick up milk or grab the Sunday paper.

VARY YOUR LOCATION, ENJOY YOUR WALKS

Walk to or from work. If you take mass transit, get off a stop or two earlier and walk the last 20 minutes to work. Or maybe you can walk all the way, and carpool home with a friend, or get picked up by your spouse.

Whatever you do, consciously think about making the walk part of your life. Now go enjoy today's 20 minutes, and have an extra glass of water afterward.

WHEN: .... AM/PM

HOW: ....

WHERE: ....

....

....

TIME: ☐

DAY 33 — 15 Minutes

So far we haven't talked much about walking speed, because it's far more important to simply create the walking habit than to go fast. However, as your body has become more accustomed to your daily walks, you're likely to have begun to walk more briskly. That's a good thing, because a bit of vigor on your walk means you'll gain more benefits.

The faster you walk, the more you tax your cardiovascular system (heart, lungs, and blood vessels) and musculoskeletal system (muscles and bones). As you already know, stressing a system causes it to adapt by making itself stronger and better able to handle the next stress. So, if you find you're actually breathing harder—not panting uncontrollably, but simply breathing enough so that it interrupts conversation—then you're stressing the heart and lungs enough to gain more benefit than if you're just casually sauntering at a nonstop conversation tempo. This is the basis of aerobic exercise—enough to gently stress the body's cardiovascular system. By the way, remember that if you are walking this briskly, an easy 3-to-5-minute stroll to warm up is a good idea.

TECHNIQUE IS THE KEY TO SPEED

If you are speeding up, make sure it comes from healthy walking technique. That means good posture (walk tall, gaze forward, no shelf-butt) and a natural stride (don't reach, let your tempo come from quicker steps). To remind yourself of that healthy posture, back up against the wall for a quick posture check—tighten those abdominals. Then walk for 15 minutes.

WHEN: _____ AM/PM

HOW: _____

WHERE: _____

_____

_____

TIME: ☐

DAY 34

10 Minutes

The muscles of your midsection are really some of the most important muscles to your walking stride. Yes, the legs do a ton of work, but your midsection provides the stable platform from which the legs generate their power. The hip flexors and thigh muscles pull your swinging leg forward and the gluteal and hamstring (butt and back of thigh) muscles provide much of the pull to get the leg back beneath you once the heel hits the ground. Both muscle groups attach across the hips to your midsection. One reason walking is such good exercise is that it involves using these large muscles in highly repetitive movements.

It's important that the abdominal muscles be strong enough to provide that stable platform, which is why you should do the posture-check exercise often. That simple act of pressing your lower back up against the wall and holding it can help strengthen the muscles of the midsection to enable them to support a healthy walking posture. A simple warm-up exercise for these muscles before your walk is a trunk rotation.

Stand with your hands on your hips and your feet shoulder-width apart, with knees very slightly bent. Now gently bend forward from the waist, then lean left, then back, then right, then forward again. Don't rush; hold each position for a count of three. And don't try to force your body into an extreme range of motion. Simply bend a comfortable amount from the waist; barely bend backward at all. The idea is to warm up the muscles of the midsection

WARM UP YOUR BODY BY ROTATING YOUR TRUNK

and get them ready to take part in your walk. Do several to the left, then several to the right.

After a few trunk rotations, head out for a 10-minute walk.

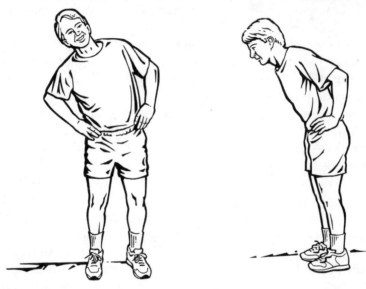

WHEN: _____ AM/PM

HOW: _____

WHERE: _____

_____

_____

TIME: [ ]

What's ideal for you may be much too fast—or too slow—for someone else. And the brisk-but-comfortable pace that feels right for you this week may feel a little slow by the end of the 90 days, as your fitness and technique improve.

Knowing your typical walking speed is valuable in two ways: First, it will satisfy your possibly intense (and certainly natural) curiosity as to how fast you really are walking. Second, it can serve as a benchmark to help measure your improving fitness. You can estimate your speed now, and compare it to what you think is a brisk pace in seven weeks—and probably find that you are walking more quickly, without even trying to.

If you would like to estimate your walking speed, measuring out a mile with the car odometer is fine, and on Day 37 we'll explain how to measure your speed quite accurately at a track. But one very simple way is to count how many steps you take each minute. As we've said, quicker steps are the key to faster walking (since your stride will only stretch so far), and your step rate increases fairly directly with your walking speed. So during your walk, just check your watch and count how many steps you take in one minute of walking. (Or, you may find it easier to count only your left or right footsteps, and then multiply by two.) Then get your rough estimate of speed from the table.

Remember that this is just an estimate, and note that taller people typically have longer legs, and so take fewer

IS THERE AN IDEAL WALKING SPEED?

Walking speed (mph)	Approximate Step Rate (steps/minute)		
	Less than 5'6" tall	5'6" to 6' tall	Taller than 6'
2.0	100–110	95–105	90–100
2.5	105–115	100–110	95–105
3.0	110–120	105–115	100–115
3.5	120–130	115–125	110–120
4.0	130–140	125–135	120–130
4.5	140–150	135–145	130–140
5.0	155–165	150–160	145–155

steps at a given speed. However, it's a myth that they will necessarily be faster walkers, since shorter walkers have less leg to swing forward on each step, and so can more easily maintain a quicker step rate.

Walk for 20 minutes today, whatever the speed. If you've followed the recommendations, with this walk you complete 90 minutes of walking this week—enough to have a real impact on your health. Keep up the good work!

WHEN: _____ AM/PM

HOW: _____

WHERE: _____

_____

_____

TIME: [ ]

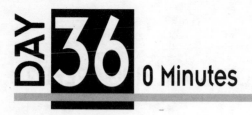

DAY 36

0 Minutes

If your exercise of choice is of modest intensity—such as the walking you've done so far—then the benefits depend very much on the regularity of the exercise. If you were working out vigorously for 45 minutes to an hour, a 3- or 4-day-per-week schedule would be logical. But if the effort is more modest, then exercise frequency is the key. You have to maintain your six-days-a-week schedule to expect your body to continue to adapt to your 15- and 20-minute walks, so that you can comfortably increase those over the next few weeks.

Keep in mind that research suggests that expending as little as 750 extra calories per week in conscious physical activity (beyond your normal daily requirements) can increase your expected lifespan measurably (an average of 1.5 years for participants of the famed Harvard Alumni study). That means an average of 125 calories a day (or roughly 30 minutes of brisk walking, your eventual goal) if spread over six days of the week. But it would require more like an hour-long workout if crammed into three days of the week.

It's also important to remember this is all about habits. Obviously you want to build good habits, like walking regularly, enjoying yourself, staying more active, eating well and drinking lots of water. But you also want to avoid bad habits, like saying it's okay to miss a day. One missed day can lead to two, then three. Next thing you know you'll be

MAINTAIN THOSE GOOD HABITS

growing your hair long and listening to rock and roll music.

So, if you missed a scheduled walk in the last six days, go for a 10-minute walk today and log it, as much as anything to prove to yourself that it is important, and that you can find the time. And to maintain the good habit, and not create a bad one.

Otherwise, check off if you practice two of your other good habits, such as skipping the fat, and eating an extra veggie (pass on the extra helping of meat loaf, and take more carrots instead), or drinking a couple of glasses of water, or being more active (park at the far edge of the mall parking lot, just for the extra walk).

WHEN: _____ AM/PM

HOW: _____

WHERE: _____

_____

_____

TIME: ☐

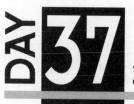

DAY 37
20 Minutes

As we have said, you don't have to be hung up about your walking speed on a day-to-day basis. But it is nice to measure improvement over time. So, if you're inclined to make an accurate estimate of your pace, taking a walk on a local high school or college track will do the trick.

Almost all outdoor tracks used for competitions are either 440 yards (exactly ¼ mile) or 400 meters (just two yards short of ¼ mile) long, so they're convenient for estimating your walking speed.

Today, if you can, or on the day of your next scheduled longer walk, go to the track. Do a few ankle circles and trunk rotations and an easy 3-to-5-minute stroll to warm up. It's cool to do these at a track—people will think you're a hotshot and you know what you're doing (which you do).

Walk the inside lane of the track, and time a half mile (two laps) or a mile (four laps). Why the inside lane? The farther out on the track you walk, the greater the distance you cover. If there are fast runners on the track, or rules prohibiting walking in the first several lanes, step into the infield, just inside the first lane, and do your four laps there. For greater accuracy, use a stopwatch, or even better, have a spouse or friend time you. (Talk about looking serious!) Don't try to walk as fast as you can, just at the same purposeful pace you usually use.

Details on assessing your time tomorrow. Today, go for a 20-minute walk, and don't forget to warm up easily for a few minutes beforehand if you're going to time yourself.

FIGURE OUT YOUR WALKING SPEED—
BUT JUST FOR LATER COMPARISON

And don't get all serious and grave if you decide to time your walk. Remember, the goal is to simply give yourself something to compare your fitness with in a few weeks.

WHEN: _____ AM/PM

HOW: _____

WHERE: _____

_____

_____

TIME: [ ]

So now you know how fast you walk a mile. Does it mean anything? Is, say, 21 minutes for a mile fast or slow? Runners often speak of their "minute-per-mile" pace, but they're already familiar with the numbers: 5 minutes per mile for a world-class marathon run, 7 minutes per mile for a quick running workout, 9 minutes per mile for a decent jog. At walking speeds, however, it's more convenient for now to convert minutes per mile into miles per hour.

Simply divide your number of minutes for a mile into 60 (or, for a half-mile time, into 30). Thus, a 20-minute mile converts into exactly 3 miles per hour. A 24-minute mile is 2.5 miles per hour, and an 18-minute mile is 3.3 miles per hour. Similarly, a 14-minute half mile equals about 2.1 miles per hour.

For the record, 3.3 mph is a typical starting speed for a healthy, fairly active person beginning a walking program. But each individual's pace is just that—individual. It's determined by your condition, weight, technique, and dozens of other factors. So don't worry about how fast

WHAT EXACTLY IS A 21-MINUTE MILE, ANYWAY?

other people typically go. It's best if you focus on your effort (noticeable but easily maintained breathing) and sound technique, and let the miles per hour come out where they may.

Enjoy a 15-minute walk today.

WHEN: AM/PM

HOW:

WHERE:

TIME:

DAY 39
20 Minutes

A while ago (Day 16) we described the basic features of a good walking shoe: a fairly low, beveled heel, a flexible forefoot, and an upper on the shoe that isn't cluttered with extra straps and layers to make it heavy.

Some people, though, need more stringent standards for their shoes. If you go through shoes really fast (say, in a couple of months or less) it's possible that you need to pay special attention to the shoes you buy.

Set your shoes on a table and look at them from behind. If the heels are crushed way inward, then you may be an overpronator, which means your foot rolls in excessively during a step. You can look for a shoe that has pronation-control features such as a stiffer material under the inside of the heel. This is called a medial post, because it's on the medial side of the foot. Many running shoes and some walking shoes have this feature. But if you go with a running shoe, be sure it has a fairly low, bevelled heel.

If you look down on your shoes from above, and it looks like the lump just behind the little toe is trying to slide off the outside of the shoe, making the upper material bulge and tear out up there, you might want to consider a shoe with more lateral support. A cross-training, court, or aerobics shoe might have a band that wraps up on the outside of the shoe to support this area.

If these problems begin to cause any discomfort it's best to see a podiatrist, or to get a referral from your doctor

TAKE CARE OF YOUR FEET—MAKE SURE YOUR SHOES DO THE JOB

right away, because you're going to be logging lots of miles with those feet. Like the 20 minutes you should head out and walk right now.

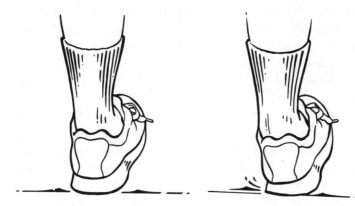

Normal   Overpronated

WHEN: AM/PM

HOW:

WHERE:

TIME:

DAY 40 — 10 Minutes

You're far along enough in your program that 10-minute walks—which may have seemed herculean a month ago—are now actually a form of rest day. But the fact that your shorter walks are feeling easy means that your longer walks are that much more critical to your overall fitness. The last three days were 15- and 20-minute walks, which ideally you are completing with near religious fervor. If, however, you have walked but fallen short of the time requirement or missed one of those days, consider making up that time today.

Remember the stress-adaptation cycle? Well, your longer walks are now the stress. With five extra minutes of walking, you're asking your heart to pump 500–1000 extra times, your leg muscles to contract for 400–700 more steps, your lungs to process 6–10 more liters of air. And your heart and leg muscles will get a little stronger, and your circulatory system a little more developed in response to that stress. But you can't skip the progressive workouts and expect to get in better shape. You have to increase the load on your system, even if in very small increments, if you want your condition to improve.

Therefore, if you skipped a 20-minute walk in the past few days, then do 20 minutes today. Or if you did 10 minutes on the 15-minute day, do 15 today—consider it a trade. The bottom line is, of course, not to get too wrapped up in the details but just to maintain the general trend of walking a little bit more each week, and being sure to do all

EASY DAYS COUNT, TOO

the longer walks since they are an important part of your fitness walking program.

Head out for a 10-minute walk (or more if you've missed something longer) and log the details.

WHEN: _____ AM/PM

HOW: _____

WHERE: _____

_____

_____

TIME: ▢

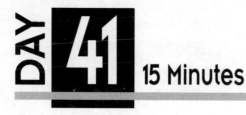

DAY 41

15 Minutes

The human body is amazing in its ability to adapt. In the most extreme case, it's able to use the nutrients we eat to reconstruct damaged tissue after an injury. The body can sometimes even make the repair stronger than the original tissue, as with some broken bones. But equally intriguing is the subtler rebuilding and strengthening that is done in response to exercise.

As you would expect, the greater the stress you put the body under, the greater the adaptation required. A broken bone may take weeks or even months to repair, but within days of a sunburn the old skin has peeled and new, healthy skin is exposed. Response to exercise can take hours or days or weeks, depending on the anatomical system you're looking at. Overdo it and make your muscles sore, and within 24 to 48 hours they'll be rebuilding themselves. Researchers have even seen the more fundamental changes associated with improved health in as little as three to six weeks if the exercise is regular enough, long enough, and intense enough. The following physiological changes have either already started, or are likely to over the next several weeks.

1. The heart muscle can grow larger and stronger, producing a lower heart rate both at rest and when exercising at a given level, because more blood is pumped with each stroke.

2. The elasticity of the arteries can increase, aiding in the circulation of blood, and the network of small capil-

HOW WE GET MORE PHYSICALLY FIT

laries that deliver blood to the muscle fibers is denser in exercised muscle.

3. Blood volume can increase, especially if you're drinking enough water, providing more red blood cells to carry oxygen to the muscles.

4. The body gets better at mobilizing and burning fat with regular exercise. You may already be experiencing some of these changes, depending on your initial fitness and how hard you've been working on your walks.

Now that you know what you're doing to your body, give it some stress with a 15-minute walk, and build some capillaries while you're at it.

WHEN: _____ AM/PM

HOW: _____

WHERE: _____

_____

_____

TIME: [ ]

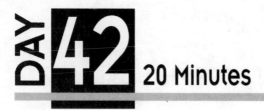

You're six weeks into the program, which suggests you're probably seeing some of the changes described yesterday. But depending on the shape you were in when you started, it's possible your body is just beginning to respond, because we've begun very gradually and with very little stress. The goal so far has been for you to see how fun walking is, how easy it is to do, and to figure out how best to make it a part of your life. Now that your walks have become a habit, we'll continue to increase the length of the workouts to gain benefits and elicit physiological changes.

There are three fundamental factors which affect the stress your body experiences during exercise: 1. how often you exercise, 2. how hard you work, and 3. how long you work. Trainers refer to these variables as F.I.T., for Frequency, Intensity, and Time. Increasing each of these factors tends to increase the stimulus to your body to rebuild and strengthen itself, as long as you don't increase to the point of injuring yourself.

The *frequency* of your workouts is pretty fixed, since you're already walking six days a week. It's nice to preserve one day off for mental and physical recovery. However, each day you get the itch to head out for a second walk, or do something else more active like take the stairs or wash the car by hand, you're increasing the frequency of your exercise, which is great.

Intensity is the next variable you can control. (We alluded to this on Day 33.) Heavier breathing suggests you're push-

WHAT TO DO TO GET MORE PHYSICALLY FIT

ing your body to a higher heart rate and greater intensity of exercise. There are many ways to do that: walking uphill, wading through water, pushing a stroller, carrying things, walking on sand. Walking faster, however, is the simplest. Just pick up the pace, take quicker steps, and you're on your way.

You're increasing the *time* of your walks at a pretty healthy rate, and though you may be comfortable walking more than the suggestions, there's no urgency to exceed them. We're suggesting increases that make good progress (you'll be up to 30 minutes before you know it) without risking discomfort.

Take a 20-minute walk. Make it as strenuous as is comfortable to strengthen your heart.

WHEN: _____ AM/PM

HOW: _____

WHERE: _____

_____

_____

TIME: ☐

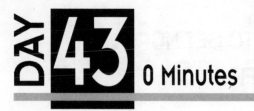

You can adjust the frequency, intensity, and time of your walks, depending on your goals. If you're most concerned about health and longevity, research suggests that 30 minutes of walking six days per week can increase your life expectancy and overall health (depending on your age and other lifestyle habits). A worthy goal, no doubt.

If your focus is on increasing your aerobic fitness and maximizing all of the training responses described on Day 40, then you could increase the intensity of two or three of your weekly walks. You might speed up to 4 mph or more, if that would elevate your heart rate and breathing noticeably (sucking wind, as some athletes call it). Such conditioning might help leave you less out of breath when carrying groceries, or less fatigued by some romping with the dog or playing with the kids.

If your goal is weight loss, adjusting the intensity of your walks can help there too, since a higher heart rate and greater oxygen consumption means that you're burning more calories (recall Day 19). But if more intense workouts leave you tired or sore the next day, you may be less likely to get out and do your full walk, and you can't afford to miss walks when you're trying to lose weight. Therefore, the best thing to do may be to increase the time you spend walking. The goal in weight loss is to burn calories, and taking long walks of moderate intensity is a great way to do that. You can even walk more frequently to crank up the calorie burn by simply getting in more short walks in a day.

BENEFITS OF INCREASING INTENSITY

When you start planning your own program, you'll be able to focus on goals like health, fitness, or weight loss simply by adjusting the frequency, intensity, and time of your walks. For now, however, focus on a day off, unless you missed a walk last week. Then either record the amount of time spent walking or check off below for doing one more active thing than usual.

WHEN: AM/PM

HOW:

WHERE:

TIME:

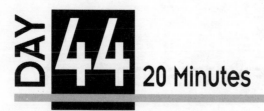

Now that you've completed six weeks of walking, your training log may have a good deal of usable information. This is a good time to check again for patterns in your personal program, especially if you've recorded things like the time of day, where you walk, and your walking companions.

Do you notice a certain day of the week on which you always miss or fall short of the goal? Maybe it's the day you carpool the kids to soccer after work, or meet your mystic, or clean your tuba. Whatever the reason, why not plan that as your day off, and walk the other six days of the week? You'll find in the end that it works out much better and reduces your stress.

Is there any specific time of day for which your comments are always positive? Do your 6:00 A.M. workouts feel great because they're a regular part of the morning routine before work, or are they sometimes cut short because you hit the snooze button an extra time? If the latter, relocate those walks to another time of day, when you'll give them their due.

Notice any ailments? Are your shins sore? If so, slow down a little, and try more ankle circles and toe points. Do you see evidence that one of your hamstrings has been getting progressively tighter over the past several workouts? Then back off, or even take a day or two off to give it a rest. Your log (and your body) may be telling you to try another activity for a couple of days. Use your log to experiment and see what works out best since your log is

TAKE A LOOK AT YOUR LOG—
ANY PATTERNS?

your best guide for developing your personal fitness program.

For most people, a log is a great motivator. Writing an unplanned "0" in your log is a letdown—even more if it happens two days in a row. So if your log simply helps you get out the door every day, that's great, even if all you record is length of walking time and nothing more.

Take a 20-minute walk today (perhaps at a time suggested by a review of your log) and record the details.

WHEN: _____ AM/PM

HOW: _____

WHERE: _____

_____

_____

TIME: ☐

Are you still thinking about healthy posture on every walk? Not only is it the basis of good walking technique, but you should be thinking about it all the time—not just when you're walking. Remember to be tall, with relaxed shoulders, and gently contract the stomach to avoid a shelf-butt. If you're picking up the pace a bit, to gradually increase the intensity and fitness benefits of your walks, remember to maintain this posture and focus on quicker steps. And, as we stated before, let the stride length come naturally—don't overstride.

One way to help with this is to focus on pushing off with your back foot. As you finish a step, think about rolling up onto your toes and pushing back on the ground as hard as you can, as if to show someone behind you the bottom of your foot. This helps extend the stride to its full length, but it extends the stride behind you rather than in front. That's good, because if you reach too far with your front foot, it tends to slow you down. (While your leg is in front of your body, you're actually pushing forward against the ground and slowing down.) That's why I emphasized (on Day 27) naturally falling into your step rather than trying to reach. A good push-off with the back foot helps.

Happily, generating more push with the foot at the end of the step means you are working the calf muscle more, which develops toned and healthy calves. The down side is that muscles often get a little stiff when they are suddenly used more than usual, so don't be surprised if your calves

MAXIMIZE THE THRUST—PUSH OFF WITH YOUR TOES

tighten up a little after you begin concentrating on pushing off. Tomorrow you'll learn an important stretch to help keep the calf healthy.

Take a 15-minute walk and concentrate on pushing off with your toes for at least the middle five minutes. Notice how this technique makes you feel like you're picking up the pace.

WHEN: _____ AM/PM

HOW: _____

WHERE: _____

_____

_____

TIME:

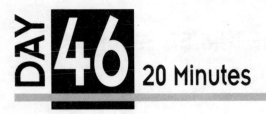

DAY 46

20 Minutes

If your calf muscles are feeling tight, here's how to take care of them. These muscles attach to the Achilles tendon, which wraps behind the heel and connects to the plantar fascia, a tough membrane on the bottom of the foot. Both of these tissues are vulnerable to irritation when the calf muscles are tight. If ignored, this can become full-fledged inflammation: tendonitis and plantar fasciitis, which can be chronic because those tissues see so much day-to-day use. The best preventative measure is to keep that whole chain of tissue as loose as possible.

Fortunately, a simple calf stretch can be done very easily while standing after every walk. Like other stretches, it should only be done after the muscles and tendons are well warmed up, perhaps best of all right after your walk. Step forward with one foot and then bend the knee of that leg so that the body begins to drop forward above that foot. You may have to use one hand to steady yourself on a wall or a chair. As the body drops forward, keep the heel of the back foot on the ground. Go down very gently, only until you feel a slight pull in the calf. There should be no pain. Hold that position for a count of 20, relaxing and breathing deeply, then slowly stand back up. Switch legs and do the other side. Remember to maintain good posture throughout this stretch. The abdominals should be tight, so that your lower back doesn't arch, and you may feel a slight stretch in the hip too, which is good. Gently repeat this stretch on each side a couple of times. You may want to

IF YOU WORK THE CALVES, STRETCH THEM

alternate these with toe points, to stretch the shin as well (but always end on the calf stretches as that's the more vulnerable tissue).

Now head out for a 20-minute walk, thinking about good push-off, and try some easy calf stretches afterward.

WHEN: _____ AM/PM

HOW: _____

WHERE: _____

_____

_____

TIME: ▢

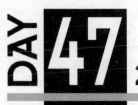

DAY 47
20 Minutes

As hard as it may be to believe, you've actually been walking for over six weeks. In general, you probably find that you look forward to your daily walks. Your body and mind have begun enjoying the myriad benefits of walking.

However, that doesn't mean it's easy to get out the door every day. Perhaps in six weeks the seasons have begun to change. Maybe the weather has gotten drearier, or it's getting dark earlier. Or it may simply be harder to find 20 minutes for a walk than it was to find 10 minutes. Here are some ideas on how to make sure you get out the door.

- **Just start to put on your walking clothes.** The mere act of putting on your most comfortable walking pants and shoes can sometimes get the adrenaline flowing in anticipation of your workout. Next thing you know, you're walking.
- **Convince yourself you're only going for five minutes.** Telling yourself that you only have to walk for five minutes (no matter how windy and wet it is outside) may be all you need to get moving. Once out the door, your elevated heart rate, increased breathing, and exercise "buzz" (those wonderful beta-endorphins) will keep you walking.
- **Tell everyone in the house you're going.** When I'm visiting home, I'm often spurred out the door by my mother saying, "What are you still doing here? I

GETTING OUT THE DOOR

thought you said you were going for a workout a half an hour ago." You bet I am, Mom.

- **Get a streak going.** Some people pride themselves on having walked every single day, continuously for years. Even though we say it's good to take one day a week off, if a streak of nonstop walking will keep you going, then give it a try. Nothing is quite as impressive as a training log that shows 100 straight days of walking. Just be sure that one or two days a week are short, easy, nontaxing strolls (like a day off to your body).

Today you walk 20 minutes, so even if you don't feel like walking, start getting dressed, decide you're only walking for a few minutes, tell everyone you're going—and keep your current 6-day streak alive.

WHEN: _____ AM/PM

HOW: _____

WHERE: _____

_____

_____

TIME: ☐

DAY 48 15 Minutes

You may have noticed that you really start breathing hard when you walk up a hill, especially if you try to maintain your pace. That's completely normal, because your leg muscles are now doing a lot more work—not just propelling you forward, but also lifting you up with each step. Thus, hills are another great way to intensify your walk and workout (see chart). The tendency is to lean forward when you're walking uphill, but you should try to maintain your healthy, upright posture as much as possible. In particular, don't lean forward too much from the waist, because that can lead to back soreness and hamstring tightness. Better lean from the ankles, if at all.

Walking Uphill:

Increased energy expenditure, as compared to walking on level ground at 3.5 mph.

Grade:	6%	10%	15%	20%
Speed:	3.5 mph	3.0 mph	2.5 mph	2.0 mph
% Increase in energy expenditure:	16%	52%	67%	70%

When walking uphill, you naturally tend to slow down because it is harder work. Slowing down a little won't keep you from increasing the exercise intensity and getting a greater calorie burn. In fact, research at the University of

ANOTHER WAY TO INTENSIFY— HEAD FOR THE HILLS

Southern California showed that in going up a 10% grade (that's 10 feet of rise for every 100 feet walked), walkers slowing from 3.5 to 3 miles an hour still saw a 52% increase in energy use. So, if your goal is to bring up the cardiovascular intensity of your walk because you want more fitness benefits, but you're not sure you can go any faster, seeking out hills is a great option. But you don't want to slow down more than necessary, so concentrate on maintaining the cadence of your steps.

For today, take a 15-minute walk and, whether hilly or flat, try to maintain good posture all the way through. Do a couple of posture-check exercises (see Day 30) after your walk to be sure.

WHEN: _____ AM/PM

HOW: _____

WHERE: _____

_____

_____

TIME: ⬜

DAY 49

20 Minutes

Today you'll finish seven weeks of walking, and be more than halfway through the 90-day program. Your body is physically responding to the exercise, and you no doubt feel the combination of reduced stress and sense of empowerment that characterizes the mental benefits of exercise. Most of all, if you've stuck with it this far, you're doing an excellent job of building a fitness walking program into your life. You're regularly doing 20-minute walks now, so you'll probably find it easy to continue adding a few more minutes a week until you reach the final goal of 30 minutes per day.

Speaking of adding minutes each week, you may notice that you will only go from 110 total minutes of suggested walking this past week to 115 next week, and 120 the week after. Usually you add 10 minutes per week ... what's happened? You're benefiting from a principle that elite athletes often use, called periodization. Varying the stress on the body is important not just on a day-to-day basis, but even on a weekly and monthly time scale. Doing the same amount of exercise all the time can lead to staleness. So, just as you mix up 10-, 15-, and 20-minute walks, you may choose to avoid that hilly loop once in a while so your body has an easier day, it's good to give yourself an easier week now and then as well.

Since these are still fairly moderate walks, simply slowing the rate of progression a bit by adding fewer minutes next week and the week after gives you a bit of a break. As you

VARIETY IS THE SPICE OF LIFE— AND WALKING

get more serious about your walking and continue to go farther and faster, or even if you just stick with a healthy, 30-minute-per-day average, remember that variety is good— by the day or the week.

Today calls for a 20-minute walk, and remember those warm-up ankle rolls and trunk rotations.

WHEN: _____ AM/PM

HOW: _____

WHERE: _____

_____

_____

TIME: [ ]

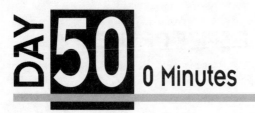

DAY 50

0 Minutes

You know that the key to maintaining a healthy weight is a combination of healthy diet and exercise. That is the best way to maintain an even calorie balance—eating the same number of calories through a healthy diet that you burn in an active lifestyle. But you may be curious about the number of calories your body burns in a day.

Actually, it's difficult to estimate the exact number of calories a person burns, because of differences in individual physiology and fitness levels, current weight, and personal lifestyle habits. But many sports nutritionists and counselors would suggest the following very rough rules of thumb for estimating your daily calorie requirements. A person requires about 10 calories per day per pound of body weight just to survive. So a 120-pound woman requires about 1200 calories a day just for her resting metabolic rate. You can then add half again to that number if you are moderately active during the day. Make the addition smaller if you literally sit at a desk and do nothing else, slightly larger if you run a day care center and chase 3-year-olds for 8 hours. So, our moderately active person adds half again to 1200, for a daily calorie requirement of 1800 calories. Now add a bit more to that caloric expenditure based on your daily walk (see Day 19 for some typical numbers).

If our hypothetical 120-pound woman walks about 3.5 miles per hour for one hour (15 minutes in the morning, 30 minutes at lunch, and 15 minutes with the dog in the

HOW MANY CALORIES IS TOO MANY?

evening), we can add another 300 calories to her daily requirements. In very simplistic terms, if she eats more than 2100 calories worth of food, she's going to gain weight over time. If she eats a bit less than 2100, she will, over time, lose weight. But that doesn't mean she should starve herself on 1000 calories a day. Small changes and steady progress are the smart route to lasting weight loss.

You can make a similar estimate for yourself, as long as you keep in mind that it is only a rough estimate, and it's just to give you an idea as to your body's daily needs. The goal here is not to turn you into a fanatic calorie counter. But knowing that there's a big difference between 2100 and 3100 calories—and knowing how far you have to walk to burn off that extra 1000—may help you to think twice before you say: "Well, it's only one donut. How much difference can that make?"

The answer is, it can put you 400 calories over your body's need for that day. And research suggests that overweight people often vastly underestimate their daily caloric intake. So, if your weight is a concern, and you become a bit more aware of what you eat because you know you're going to be out there burning it off tomorrow, that's great. Today's a day off, so check if you make up for any missed days this week, and drink some extra water (0 calories), too.

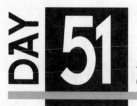

DAY 51

25 Minutes

Today you're going for a 25-minute walk. It may be your first walk for that amount of time, and as your walks get longer and accumulate more total minutes each week, they begin to burn significant numbers of calories. Now that you've walked for over seven weeks, you may have begun to build some muscle. Good things are happening in those muscles, even down at the cellular level. As you do more work in the coming weeks, the cells of those working muscles should develop more mitochondria, the energy production sites in the cells. Then they become better calorie burners, even when you're not walking.

That's more reason to keep giving your body good fuel: less fat, more fruit and vegetables, more whole grains and legumes, and lots of water. Think about what that combination of healthy diet going into an exercising body can do.

Imagine identical twins with identical lifestyles and jobs. They each get a 15-minute break in the morning, and another 10 minutes in the afternoon. One lounges at her desk with coffee and a donut in the morning, then has a candy bar or a cookie for "quick energy" in the afternoon. The other twin has juice, whole grain cereal with 1% milk and a banana for breakfast before work, takes a brisk 15-minute stroll during the first break, a 10-minute walk during the afternoon, drinks a big bottle of water and eats a piece of fruit afterward. Once a week she skips the afternoon walk to join her sister for a cookie—remember, we're not talking total deprivation here.

MORE ABOUT DIET—KEEP WATCHING THE BASICS

All other things being equal, which twin do you think will live longer? Statistics agree with your intuition and say the second is bound for a longer life. Simply 25 minutes more of daily activity can improve her life expectancy. The bottom line is that all the little things—like how you approach a coffee break—make a difference.

Focus on how you approach your "free" time today, then take a brisk 25-minute walk, and have plenty of water and a healthy snack afterward.

WHEN: _____ AM/PM

HOW: _____

WHERE: _____

_____

_____

TIME: □

DAY 52 15 Minutes

The muscles of the back of your body do a lot while you're walking. They all work to pull your leg back on each stride. It's the muscles of the lower back, the gluteals (your butt), and the hamstring (back of the thigh) that especially do the job when your heel first strikes the ground. So, it's not uncommon for those muscles to suffer a bit when you increase the walking workload. The more you walk, the more briskly you walk, and the more you walk on hills, the more likely those muscles are to tighten up. So it's appropriate to very gently stretch them after your walk.

Remember that it's important to stretch only when muscles are warm and compliant. So, although you do your warm-ups (ankle circles, trunk rotations) before you walk, do your stretching after warm-up exercises and a few minutes of walking. Or, better yet, after your walk altogether.

A hamstring stretch is like trying to touch your toes without actually trying to touch your toes. Stand with your feet about one foot apart and your knees very slightly bent. Easily bend forward from the waist, letting your head and arms hang loosely. Relax, breathing very easily. Just hang in that position for a slow 20 count, and then slowly stand back up. Relax for a moment and then repeat that stretch two more times. It's very simple, but it will tend to stretch all the right muscles: the back, lower back, gluteals, and hamstrings.

STRETCH THE HAMSTRINGS—GENTLY

Now enjoy your 15-minute walk, and afterward gently stretch your hamstrings and remember to do some calf stretches, as well.

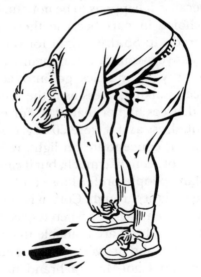

WHEN: _____ AM/PM

HOW: _____

WHERE: _____

_____

_____

TIME: ☐

DAY 53
20 Minutes

To dress properly for walking, you have to dress for the season. That's because walking is a year-round activity. It is unnecessary to give up your walk just because of a little rain or wind, or because it happens to be hot out. Walking is the exercise of choice in part because there are few good excuses not to do it. So dress right for the weather, and enjoy your walks year-round. Just remember, you'll be getting warmer as your muscles go into action. So, for moderate-paced walking, dress as if the temperature was about 10–15 degrees higher than it is. For example, if it's 50 degrees out, dress as if it were 60 degrees.

In the summer, concentrate on light, reflective colors. Doing this may not seem like much, but it can really make a difference. Many people prefer loose and airy clothes, so that the air flows right through. Cotton is comfortable, but less so when you sweat because when it gets wet, it tends to stay wet. Synthetic fabrics are available that wick moisture away from your skin and dry very quickly. Materials such as polypropylene and Cool-Max (a brand name from Du-Pont) do this, and are available in undergarments as well as in jerseys and tights.

Interestingly enough, the same materials that wick away sweat in summer are also the logical start to dressing properly in winter. The key is to build layers from your skin outward, beginning with a comfortable close-to-the-skin layer, followed by some insulators, then a shell to protect from the elements.

WALKING CLOTHING—COMFORT IS THE KEY

Tights, by the way, are a topic in and of themselves. Not only can they be an immense fashion statement (my personal preference is the zebra stripe), but they also provide some relief if you have problems with chafing legs. Another remedy for chafing (legs, armpits, or anywhere), often bothersome in the heat and sweat of summer, is some Vaseline right on the problem area.

More on clothing tomorrow. Today, stay comfortable and climate-controlled on your 20-minute walk. And drink extra water if it is warm—that's your first line of defense against heat.

WHEN: _____ AM/PM

HOW: _____

WHERE: _____

_____

_____

TIME: ☐

DAY 54
15 Minutes

You build layers when dressing for the winter, because that gives you adjustability. If you've overdressed, you can open up or remove a layer. If you get cold, zip up or add a layer.

Start with an inner layer of synthetic wicking materials like the ones mentioned yesterday, or with silk long-johns, the natural version of the new synthetics.

For the insulating layer, you're best off with materials that insulate even when wet. Wool is the old standby (I still have a favorite wool sweater), but newer high-tech fleece materials have the same insulating value with a fraction of the weight of wool. Some even use recycled plastic as a raw material. Most have zippers so that you can adjust them if you warm up or cool down during the walk.

Your outer layer should be a wind stopper and water resistant. The old standard is a simple, nylon-coated jacket. It can keep the wind and moisture out, but it also keeps sweat in. In the last decade, advanced outer-garment fabrics such as Gore-Tex and comparable materials that can breathe out water vapor, but still protect you from the elements, have become widely available. If you live in a northern climate, they may be worth the investment.

WALKING IN WINTER? THINK IN LAYERS

The bottom line is to simply dress comfortably enough that you can enjoy your walks and never skip a day. In that spirit, head out for 15 minutes now, and remember to do some hamstring and calf stretches afterward.

WHEN: _____ AM/PM

HOW: _____

WHERE: _____

_____

_____

TIME: ☐

DAY 55
20 Minutes

We can't overemphasize how important a relaxed, comfortable technique is to your walking. It's the key to your improvement, and the key to speed. Even as you speed up, stick with the basics that we've already talked about in technique.

One way to maintain a healthy, natural walking posture is to avoid carrying things while you walk. Even something as small as a radio or tape player for headphones, since it's carried in one hand, may throw a bit of asymmetry into your stride. Better to clip it onto your belt or waistband if at all possible. Speaking of headphones, make sure that you are extra alert if you do choose to wear them. The fact that you have slightly reduced hearing when wearing headphones means you may be less aware of traffic, cyclists, or other pedestrians coming up from behind. Be especially cautious if you choose to wear them when walking in a new or unfamiliar area.

If you do want to carry things while walking, it is probably best to carry them in a knapsack worn properly over both shoulders. Research at Auburn University on young walkers indicated that carrying gym bags or knapsacks slung over one shoulder tended to significantly twist the shoulders and spine, while those stresses were greatly reduced when the same amount of weight was worn in a backpack over both shoulders. So, don't do the cool and casual toss of a bag over one shoulder if you're walking to work, or to the store for errands. Instead, give your neck,

THINK ABOUT TECHNIQUE—SPEED
WILL FOLLOW

shoulders, and back a break, and distribute the load of all those files or that gallon of milk in a knapsack.

Now, consider taking yourself through the full walking routine that you've learned so far, if you don't already do this regularly. Warm up with ankle circles on both feet, trunk rotations, and a few posture checks to lock in that feeling before your walk. Start easily, then cruise through a 20-minute walk with perfect posture. Finish up with some toe points, calf stretches, and hamstring stretches. Take your time with these—relax and count out the easy 20 seconds in the hold position, and do a couple of each of these three stretches to really get some benefit. And then notice how long the whole thing took. Less than 30 minutes?

WHEN: _____ AM/PM

HOW: _____

WHERE: _____

_____

_____

TIME:

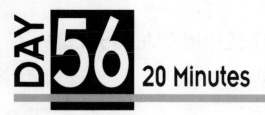

DAY 56 20 Minutes

With today's 20-minute walk, you'll complete eight weeks of walking. That's a great accomplishment in itself, worthy of congratulations. But even more than that, you've learned a great deal about maintaining your overall health and well-being. Not just how many minutes to walk, or proper technique, but other exercises and stretches you can do, plus how to eat intelligently, and the importance of drinking plenty of water.

You may be checking off your training log to simply mark your progress, or you may revel in each daily victory by recording every detail of every walk. The more you do for your overall health and fitness, the more you should congratulate yourself on your progress.

We've added a line ("other") where you can account for all the things you do around your walk, including before and after. Start with your ankle circles and trunk rotations. Then, of course, you can record the details of your walk, and afterward, record whether you did calf stretches, toe points, or hamstring stretches. Include whether you've done your posture check up against the wall, an exercise you should be doing every time you think of it. The list becomes a daily testimony to your improving fitness.

Realistically, should you expect to do all those exercises every day? Well, the most important thing by far is that you do your walk. But you certainly *can* do the supplemental stretches and strengtheners each day. Yesterday's walk, if you went through the whole routine, proved that supple-

LOG IT ALL—YOU'LL FEEL GREAT

ments add only 5 or 10 minutes to a session. If you do them, get in the habit of recording it. It might help you to trace potential problems. For example, if you do a lot of walking on hills, and notice that your hamstring has been very tight, you might look back in your log and see that you haven't stretched in over a week.

For now, head out for a 20-minute walk, and record any and all details that you like.

WHEN: AM/PM
_____

HOW:
_____

WHERE:
_____

OTHER:
_____

_____

TIME: □

DAY 57

0 Minutes

You may have heard of T.H.R., a term used by exercise physiologists and instructors. It stands for *target heart rate,* and refers to the appropriate range for your heart rate during exercise.

The premise is that if your heart rate is too low when you're exercising, you don't gain much cardiovascular benefit because there's not ample stress to your cardiovascular system. Your heart would barely know the difference between you taking your daily walk and sitting around watching television. And remember the stress-adaptation principle; the less the stress the less your system will adapt.

On the other hand, if your heart rate is too high during exercise, you'll fatigue within minutes, before you have a chance to do any work. Your heart would think it's just another dash up the stairs because the elevator's broken.

Experts calculate the target heart rate range in terms of *maximum heart rate,* or M.H.R. (the highest heart rate your body can safely reach). The original recommendations, based on research at the Cooper Clinic for Aerobic Research and other laboratories, indicated that exercising at a heart rate between 60 and 80 percent of your maximum heart rate was the most efficient way to cause an increase in fitness over time, while being safe and sustainable. So, if you hear someone say, "Your T.H.R. is sixty to eighty percent of your M.H.R.," that's all they mean.

More recent research indicates that regular activity at

DEFINING T.H.R.

lower heart rates, like 50 and perhaps even 40 percent of maximum, also has beneficial effects on health and longevity. But it's not likely to make your cardiovascular system much more able to sustain hard work.

We'll continue with T.H.R. tomorrow, but since today is a day off, check off for doing something active other than walking. Go golfing, or parachute jumping, or scuba diving, or just chase the dog around the yard for a half hour. Of course, if you're making up for a missed day, mark that in your log.

WHEN: AM/PM

HOW:

WHERE:

OTHER:

TIME:

DAY 58
25 Minutes

The best way to determine your target heart rate is to get a stress test from your doctor. That test on the treadmill (briefly described on Day 10) allows the doctor to look very closely at how your system responds to exercise. He or she can accurately estimate your maximum heart rate from the test, and can then prescribe target heart rates (typically 60 to 80 percent) for exercise. The doctor can also modify the prescription if he or she sees anything unusual during the test, such as an irregular heartbeat or unexpected changes in blood pressure.

But not everyone needs or takes a stress test. So, researchers also determined a formula you can use to approximate your maximum heart rate without getting it measured on a treadmill. The average maximum heart rate for a 20-year-old is about 200 beats per minute. Your maximum heart rate drops about one beat per year as you get older (the heart, like other muscles, loses some strength with age). So the equation is simple: 220 minus your age equals your maximum heart rate. You can then take 60 percent and 80 percent of that number and have a rough estimate of the proper range for your target heart rate.

For overweight people, or unfit people, or extremely fit people, however, that estimate may be inaccurate. A very fit woman, for example, might have a significantly higher maximum heart rate than the equation produces, and so may end up with a target range that is too low to even make her breathe hard. On the other hand, researchers have

DETERMINING T.H.R.

suggested that obese people may begin with a somewhat lower maximum heart rate, but it may drop more slowly: only one beat in every two years. So for these people, the equation may be: 220 minus one half your age equals maximum heart rate. The point is, there's just not a very simple answer to this.

For now, go out and do a brisk, purposeful 25-minute walk. More on heart rates tomorrow.

WHEN: _____ AM/PM

HOW: _____

WHERE: _____

OTHER: _____

_____

TIME: [ ]

If you or your doctor have calculated your target heart rate, what can be done with that number? Well, if you're exercising below that range, you're still doing good things for your muscles and bones and blood chemistry, but perhaps not as much as you could to strengthen your heart and improve its efficiency. Speeding up a little bit could move you into your target range with less effort than you might imagine.

Test your T.H.R. by stopping at the midpoint of your walk and taking your pulse for a minute. This is done most simply by placing your first two fingers on the inside of your opposite wrist, or gently on your neck, beside your Adam's apple. Count the heartbeats for 15 seconds, then multiply by four. When you continue walking, adjust your speed accordingly. If you needed to speed up to reach your T.H.R., stop again in five minutes for another pulse check to see if you've gotten there. If over time you find that knowing your heart rate helps you, you might invest in an electronic heart rate monitor. That's a device that's worn around your chest that measures your heart rate and transmits it to a small watch on your wrist. You can then watch your heart rate, and speed up if it gets below 60% of your maximum, and slow down if it gets above 80% of your maximum. The fancy monitors even have an alarm built in so that you can enter the values for 60% and 80% of your maximum heart rate, and they will beep if you go outside the range.

TRYING TO REACH YOUR T.H.R.

Actually, in following this program, you've already been trying to reach your T.H.R.

Until now, you've used the layman's test, based roughly on what physiologists call your rate of perceived exertion (R.P.E.). That is, how hard you *feel* you're working. But rather than give you a number, say 12 out of 20 on the R.P.E. scale, we've described it qualitatively. We recommend a purposeful walk, which is brisk and causes noticeable breathing, but not gasping for breath. That's because when you're breathing noticeably, you're probably above 60 percent of your maximum heart rate, but if you avoid getting out of breath, you're still below 80 percent.

So for now, head out for a nice brisk 15-minute walk, notice your breathing, but no panting, and enjoy yourself.

WHEN: _____ AM/PM

HOW: _____

WHERE: _____

OTHER: _____

_____

TIME: □

DAY 60
20 Minutes

Walking is practically an injury-free activity. Because of the low impact and the natural range of motion, walkers experience few problems. But by its nature, exercise is a stress to your system and this means you can occasionally stress too much.

The most common ailments experienced by walkers are called overuse injuries. They are usually the result of trying to increase the frequency, intensity, or time (or some combination) of your walking too rapidly. The most vulnerable tissues can suffer damage because you're applying stress more rapidly than your body can compensate for it. And although you should definitely see your doctor if any pain persists or comes on very acutely, it is worth knowing the basics of self-care. Then, whether it's some tendonitis in the shin or a slightly turned ankle from stepping off a curb, you will know the first steps for treatment.

The basic prescription is to start with R.I.C.E. That acronym, used by athletic trainers, stands for *rest, ice, compression,* and *elevation.* This recommendation is especially appropriate for walking because most walking injuries involve inflammation, and they'll respond to very conservative or simple treatment, which is often the case when muscles are overused.

Rest is the most important because you have to let the tissues heal themselves. If you twist an ankle in the first five minutes of a 25-minute walk, don't be a hero. Go home and rest it! This is not the Olympic 50K racewalk. A real

IN CASE OF PROBLEMS, REMEMBER R.I.C.E.

injury is one of the few good excuses for missing a workout. In the long run, if you don't let an injury heal, you could end up missing far more days because of complications than if you simply take a few days off when it first occurs. So take a break, and let the injury heal. Try some alternatives—swimming, riding a bike, raking leaves—anything that doesn't stress the injured area.

More on I, C, and E tomorrow. Today, stay injury free with a 20-minute walk and record the details.

WHEN: _____ AM/PM

HOW: _____

WHERE: _____

OTHER: _____

_____

TIME: [ ]

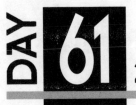

DAY 61 — 20 Minutes

Since many injuries to walkers are either simple soreness or overuse problems, the "I" in R.I.C.E. is critical. Ice is the first course of action for most athletic injuries because it reduces inflammation right away. Another reason it appears so beneficial is because it increases blood flow to the area, which brings more nutrients and removes waste and damaged tissue.

Put crushed ice in a plastic bag and hold it on the injured area or wrap it in place with an elastic bandage. You can leave it there for a maximum of 15 minutes, but obviously should pull it off if the area turns white or begins to burn, since those are early signs of frostbite. Another option is to put small paper cups full of water in the freezer. Once the water is frozen, peel away the upper part of the cup, use the bottom of the cup as a holder and massage the ice directly on the injured area. This is ideal for calf or Achilles tendon soreness because the ice melts to the shape of your leg there. But you have to be extra careful when you're applying ice directly to the skin. Only keep it on for a maximum of 10 minutes and watch out for signs of frostbite. After the area warms up (you can use a warm washcloth to facilitate this), you can apply the ice again in the same manner.

The "C" and "E" stand for compression and elevation. Elevating the injured area above the heart helps reduce swelling (for example, sleep with a twisted ankle on a pillow) as fluid can drain toward the body, for elimination.

THE REST OF THE FORMULA

Compression or wrapping it in an elastic bandage after icing (but not too tight) also applies pressure to reduce inflammation. Also note that over-the-counter painkillers containing aspirin, ibuprofen, and naproxen sodium (available in various brand-name products) are also effective anti-inflammatory agents. But use them only as directed, and see a doctor if your problem persists for more than a few days.

Now that you're an injury expert, walk for 20 minutes and be on the alert for injured runners, so you can offer them advice!

WHEN: AM/PM

HOW:

WHERE:

OTHER:

TIME:

DAY 62
15 Minutes

Since the detailed discourse on exercise heart rate, you may be asking, "Gee, how have I been doing? Am I walking fast enough? Am I really getting any benefit if I never take my heart rate?"

The answer is an unequivocal yes! Remember that the benefits from exercise come in degrees. By simply being more active (and you've been engaging in 15 to 25 minutes of activity nearly every day for the last two months), you'll see benefits such as reduced risk of heart disease and hypertension. The heart-rate discussion really focuses on improving your fitness as well as your health. This is worth attaining over time, but doesn't have to happen all at once.

Improved conditioning is a worthy goal because not only do the disease risks drop even further with greater aerobic fitness, but daily life gets better as well. If you can improve your cardiovascular fitness, you're not out of breath when you run upstairs, or carry a child or hustle after a bus. If you continue with the stretches and exercises, you'll also improve your muscle flexibility and tone. Then even movements such as the lifts, bends, and twists of daily life will get easier, and your fitness will help prevent such common ailments as back and shoulder pain.

If you do want to make a more conscious effort regarding your exercise heart rate, do it by picking up your walking pace on shorter days, like today. You don't have to have a heart-rate monitor or even stop to take your pulse. Just monitor your perceived exertion. Ask yourself: Is this

HAVE YOU BEEN THINKING
ABOUT T.H.R.?

really a brisk, purposeful walk? Do I notice increased breathing? Am I gasping or panting? But if you haven't been experimenting with brisk walking previously, don't start all at once. Try it only two or three times per week, and add it gradually to your program.

Think about maintaining your natural technique and taking quicker steps. Start with a 3-to-5-minute easy stroll to warm up, then increase your step rate until you notice you're breathing deeply and fully, but stay well below the gasp-and-wheeze zone that will just cut your walk short. Take a 15-minute walk today, and pick up the tempo if you feel like it. Then record the details below.

WHEN: AM/PM

HOW:

WHERE:

OTHER:

TIME:

DAY 63 25 Minutes

With today's 25-minute walk, you'll accumulate over two hours of fitness walking this week. Quite an accomplishment, considering you started only nine weeks ago. More importantly, if you've followed the program closely, you've done it without injury or frustration because you've built good habits slowly and gradually over the last nine weeks.

To keep seeing progress, you should continue to follow those good habits. First, keep walking six days a week, no matter what.

Next, you should be alternating your harder and easier efforts. Whether those harder efforts involve going faster, or walking on hills, carrying a child in a backpack, or simply taking longer walks, use your breathing and how you feel as your guide. That kind of variety is going to keep your fitness program from becoming a boring routine.

Third, you should be maintaining your good posture and your quick steps, always thinking about a solid, natural technique.

Fourth, you should always be thinking about eating well and drinking lots of water.

Fifth, you should be starting your walk with a few minutes of easy warm-up strolling. You should be using the warm-up exercises before and the stretches after your walk, especially if you notice particular problem areas such as sore or tight muscles.

ACCUMULATING TWO HOURS OF EXERCISE THIS WEEK

Keep up the great habits, go out for a 25-minute walk, and congratulate yourself on two hours of exercise this week! Great job!!

WHEN: _____ AM/PM

HOW: _____

WHERE: _____

OTHER: _____

_____

TIME: [ ]

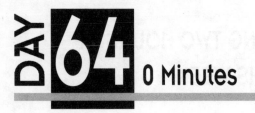

DAY 64
0 Minutes

Rugged terrain can be fun for walking, especially when there is good scenery. In fact, there are lots of options for good weekend walks, and rugged terrain is just one of them.

The key is to begin to explore new walking areas whenever you have time. Now that you're getting more fit, your legs can take you places you might not have considered going before. Look in the local area for nature preserves or protected areas, especially along rivers and lakes. You may be near a state or national park or forest. In fact, rangers in national parks often say that some of the best sights are just a short walk away from the roads and parking lots, but they are missed by the majority of visitors who never leave their cars. Now that you're a walker, you can go seek out those sights with an easy 20- or 30-minute jaunt.

Most parks and preserves provide trail maps, too. Get in the habit of using these, since they often list estimated walking times for the various trails. The guidebooks available in most bookstores are also great tools for finding new walking venues. They range from trekking guides for the most rugged territory in the country for those ready to venture into true mountaineering, to simple "where to" books, like *50 Hikes in Eastern Massachusetts*, or *20 Great Urban Walks in Seattle*. Finally, local or regional outing or hiking clubs may publish their own guides, such as the Appalachian Mountain Club's extensive trail guides for the northeastern U.S.

WEEKEND WALKS ARE GREAT FOR A CHANGE OF SCENERY

Search out resources, speak to other walkers, and take advantage of your ever-improving fitness to explore on the weekends. Since today is a day off, check off if sometime during the past week you explored and took a walk somewhere different, or if you take 15 minutes today to find a guidebook of walks in your area.

WHEN: _____ AM/PM

HOW: _____

WHERE: _____

OTHER: _____

_____

DAY 65

25 Minutes

Once you begin vigorous hikes, you may experience sore muscles. The best thing to do would be to take a rest, right? Wrong! The best thing to do would be to go for a nice, easy walk the next day.

If you hike over rugged terrain, it's possible that your calves will be sore afterward. That's because you've been lifting your body, and working hard with those muscles. It's also possible that your quadriceps—the big muscle group on the front of your thigh—will be sore. That's also from lifting your body up the hill. But the quadriceps also get tight and sore from walking downhill.

Normally our muscles undergo what are called concentric contractions. That means the muscle is shortening when it does work. For example, your bicep, the muscle on your upper arm, shortens when you bend your elbow. Watch it and see. However, when you're walking downhill, the quadriceps undergo an eccentric contraction. That means they're actually being stretched and lengthened while they are working because they're controlling your descent and keeping you from falling over forward.

In general, a muscle gets sore when you ask it to do more than it is accustomed to doing. But research suggests that the soreness is even worse if eccentric contractions are involved. That's why your legs can be very sore after a day of jumping around during a family Frisbee or softball game. If you moved sideways and leapt in the air a lot, a lot of

TAKE A RECOVERY WALK IF
YOU'RE SORE

eccentric muscle contractions occurred during your stops and landings.

More on muscle care tomorrow. For now, take your 25-minute walk, unless this is a recovery day from a vigorous hike or a vicious three-hour lawn volleyball tournament. In that case just go out for a 10- or 15-minute easy walk, to loosen up.

WHEN: _____ AM/PM

HOW: _____

WHERE: _____

OTHER: _____

_____

TIME: [ ]

DAY 66

20 Minutes

Yesterday, we talked about muscles being sore after hard work, unfamiliar exercise, or eccentric muscle contractions, such as walking downhill or jumping up and down.

Getting out and walking loosens up the sore muscle by elevating its temperature, making the tissue more compliant and able to regain its full range of motion. This is the best cure for muscle soreness. Gentle exercise also increases blood flow to the area, which is beneficial because it brings nutrients and oxygen for muscle repair, and helps to remove damaged tissue.

When you walk to relieve soreness, start very easily. Do some ankle circles and trunk rotations and then proceed slowly for the first five minutes. After 10 minutes or so of walking you'll find you're feeling much better. It's also valuable to stretch after your walk. You already know how to stretch your calves and hamstrings (Days 46 and 52) and to use toe points for your shins (Day 15). Do a few of each of these.

You can also add a thigh stretch. Stand on one foot (you may have to hold onto something for balance) and lift the other foot behind you. Reach behind yourself with the opposite hand and grab the toes. Very gently pull the toes up toward your butt, but stop as soon as you feel any pull in the thigh. Your heel doesn't have to reach your butt, and you shouldn't feel any discomfort. Hold this position for 20 seconds, breathing easily and deeply, then release your foot and do the other side. Repeat both sides one more time.

Take a refreshing 20-minute walk, and afterward try some easy thigh stretches on both legs.

DON'T LET SORE MUSCLES STIFFEN—
WALK AND STRETCH

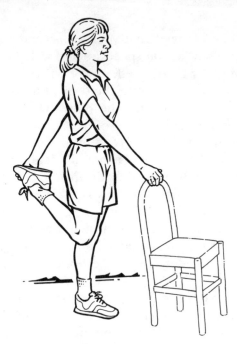

WHEN: _____ AM/PM

HOW: _____

WHERE: _____

OTHER: _____

_____

TIME: [ ]

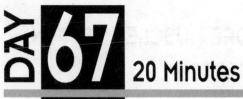

DAY 67

20 Minutes

Have you ever noticed that your arms tend to naturally bend at the elbow as you speed up and walk faster? If you haven't noticed it on yourself, imagine this for a moment. Think of kids running along the deck at a pool. The lifeguard's whistle squeals and she yells, "Hey, you kids, no running! Walk over there!"

What do they do? They break into a walk. A really *fast* walk. A quick-stepping, bent-arm walk. It almost looks like racewalking. And why do they do that? Certainly nobody has ever told them that's the way to walk the fastest. They're just trying to get somewhere quickly, without running. They take very quick steps because of the natural limit on stride length which we've talked about. Quicker steps are simply more efficient. That's the reason for bending the arms, too.

The arms and legs must swing synchronistically. And the arm will swing more quickly if bent at the elbow. Try it while standing still. Or consider the pendulum on a grandfather clock. When the clock is running slowly, you can fix this by moving the weight upward; the pendulum is shortened so that it swings more quickly. Bending the elbow effectively does the same thing—shortening the pendulum of the human arm so that it can swing more rapidly.

So, there's no reason to hold the arms straight and march like a tin soldier. Nor do you have to force them to bend at the elbow. Simply allow the arms to bend naturally as you pick up speed, and you'll be fine. Today on your 20-

USING YOUR ARMS AS AN ALLY IN FITNESS

minute walk, concentrate on walking more briskly during the middle 10 minutes and notice what your arms do. Do they tend to bend a little bit as you really speed up? It's only natural.

WHEN: AM/PM

HOW:

WHERE:

OTHER:

TIME:

You now have a fairly complete lower-body stretching routine for after your walk. You don't have to use it after every workout, but if you ever feel some tightness or stiffness, it's comforting to know you have exercises for both the front and back muscles of your entire lower body.

You can use the calf stretch for the back of the lower leg, and the toe point for the shin. In the upper part of the leg, you can stretch the hamstring with an easy forward bend at the waist and the front of the thigh by gently lifting your heel behind your body, and an easy trunk rotation will stretch the midsection. Just go slowly and hold each position for a 5 or 10 count to get a bit of a stretch.

The last thing we should add is a simple shoulder stretch for the upper back and shoulder girdle. As you use your arms more, this area may stiffen a bit, and this is the perfect stretch for that ailment. Reach straight up with your hand, as if trying to touch the ceiling. Then bend the elbow of that arm and drop that hand behind your head and neck, leaving the elbow pointing toward the ceiling. Now very gently reach up behind your head with the other hand and pull that elbow across above your head very slowly. Stop as soon as you feel a very gentle pull in the shoulder, armpit, or back, or if there is any discomfort. Hold for a

STRETCH THE SHOULDERS, TOO

count of 20, breathing easily and deeply, then slowly release and relax. Repeat on the other side, and do once more on each side.

Cruise through your 25-minute walk, and try some easy shoulder and thigh stretches afterward.

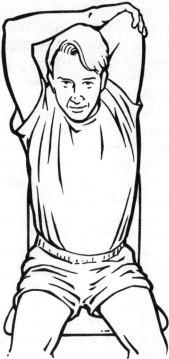

WHEN: _____ AM/PM

HOW: _____

WHERE: _____

OTHER: _____

_____

TIME: ☐

DAY 69
20 Minutes

Your arm swing during the walking stride can be more than just an accident of nature. You can intentionally use arm movement to broaden your workout. By getting the arms more involved, you can help tone the upper-body muscles more. But you can also increase the calorie burn of the exercise, because you're involving more muscles. Research shows that even if you don't speed up, the calorie burn tends to increase if the arms are pumped more vigorously.

You can really intensify your workout if you use bent arm technique to help you walk faster, because a faster walk is a more calorie-consuming walk (recall Day 19). However, it should not be an exaggerated pumping action. At the most, the elbow should only bend 90 degrees. The natural arc that your hand should trace is fairly small: from your waistband above the hip (no farther back), to in front of your sternum, about 6 to 12 inches in front of the chest. The hands should come to the center line but not any farther across the body, and the elbows should stay in. Letting the elbows flap out to the side, called chicken-winging, is not only inefficient but it looks silly.

YOUR ARMS CAN BROADEN
YOUR WORKOUT

Start your 20-minute walk today by easily walking for 5 to
10 minutes. Then consider consciously bending your arms
at the elbow for a 2-minute pick-up in tempo; relax for a
few minutes, and then pick it up again for two minutes.
When you bend your arms like that, walking truly becomes
a total body exercise. Continue walking for a total of 20
minutes.

WHEN: _____ AM/PM

HOW: _____

WHERE: _____

OTHER: _____

_____

TIME:

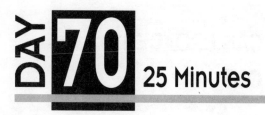

As you get more fit and walk more briskly, even if you don't consciously bend your arms at the elbows, your arms and shoulders are going to get more involved in your walking stride. They'll swing more vigorously, if only to keep up with the quicker-stepping legs. So, it's logical to add a simple upper body warm-up to those you already have.

Remember, none of the warm-up exercises, or stretches for that matter, are mandatory. You should try them when we introduce them, so that if something is stiff or tight before you walk you can take a minute to use the warm-up and gently prepare that area for the exercise. You can also gently stretch any problem areas after your walk. And you can record in your log if something has been stiff or sore, to remind you to warm it up the next day.

For the arms, shoulders, and back, try this. Hold your arms straight out to the sides. Begin tracing slow, backward circles with your hand, only six inches in diameter at first. After five or six, slowly begin to expand the circles until they're two feet in diameter and you're making nice big loops with your hands and arms. Stop and rest for a second, then start with small circles in the forward direction, again starting at six inches and increasing to two-foot-diameter circles. Do this a couple of times, until your arms and shoulders feel nice and warm.

Do some arm circles, ankle circles, and trunk rotations to warm up today, and then do a toasty 25-minute walk.

WARM THEM UP, IF YOU'RE GOING TO USE THEM

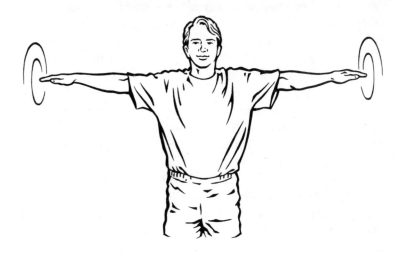

WHEN: _____ AM/PM

HOW: _____

WHERE: _____

OTHER: _____

_____

DAY 71
0 Minutes

You've probably just about hit the saturation point on all the information you've been absorbing: warm-ups, stretches, exercises afterward, brisk walking, proper technique. And you're possibly wondering, how can I do it all? What happened to good old Day 20, when we were just happy to get out and do an easy 15-minute walk? Well, don't panic. You don't have to do it all—but doing it all is probably easier than you think.

Remember, the idea in learning all those extra exercises was not that you *have* to do them, but that it is valuable for you to know them should you need them. If you wake up one morning and your calf is a bit sore you can do some extra ankle circles before your walk. Afterward you can do some gentle calf stretches. If playing tennis or hanging wallpaper yesterday left some shoulder soreness, those easy arm circles before your walk and gentle shoulder stretches afterward should help. These are the ways that these exercises and a fitness walking program contribute to your overall well-being.

The other side of the coin is that you now have a very simple total body exercise routine that you could easily fit into 45 minutes, including a 30-minute walk. For example, start with 5 to 10 ankle circles on each foot, 5 to 8 trunk rotations in each direction, and 10 to 20 arm circles in each direction, and you've spent less than five minutes warming up. Take your 30-minute walk. Finish with a set of 3 or 4 posture checks up against the wall. Then spend two

MAKING TIME FOR FITNESS

minutes each on toe points, calf, hamstring, thigh, and shoulder stretches. All of that fits in 45 minutes. The best part is that with all of this you are strengthening and toning the muscles you are using, as well as warming them up and keeping them flexible. Doing that just three days a week could really broaden some of the toning and strengthening effect of your walking program.

Today's a day off. But to convince yourself of the short amount of time needed for this entire program, go through the routine we described just once. From the first ankle circle to the last shoulder stretch, you'll probably spend only 15 to 20 minutes. Then check it off.

WHEN: _____ AM/PM

HOW: _____

WHERE: _____

OTHER: _____

_____

TIME: ☐

DAY 72 30 Minutes

Today you are walking 30 minutes, and that's the maximum amount of walking time built into the program outlined by this book. If this is your first 30-minute venture, congratulations! Only by virtue of patient building of your fitness routine have you gotten to the point where you can go out for a 30-minute walk and cover the distance with ease.

The ideal is for you to do this continuously and briskly. As we said when discussing target heart rate, to have an impact on your fitness you have to engage in continuous, purposeful aerobic activity that elevates your heart rate somewhat and that you maintain for more than 20 minutes. (Fitness, remember, is the ability to chase the dog or dash up the stairs and not get exhausted.)

To maintain health, it appears that getting in a regular 30 minutes of activity is still important, but it may not be as important for it to be continuous activity. This is still an area in which physiologists and physicians are constantly doing research to improve our understanding of what elicits a response in the body. But it seems to be true that as long as your bouts of exercise are 10 minutes or longer, and you still have a total of 30 minutes of activity per day, there are still substantial rewards. And the activity should still be purposeful—a brisk walk that allows you to notice you are breathing—but it could be a 15-minute walk to the bus in the morning and a 15-minute walk back home in the afternoon. Or you might walk 10 minutes at lunch and 20 minutes again in the evening after dinner.

YOU'RE UP TO TARGET TIME

Your best bet is to try for a continuous walk whenever possible. But if occasionally you have to break it up, then do so, and know that it's still doing plenty of good.

Head out for a 30-minute walk, ideally all at once, and congratulate yourself with every step on what a wonderful job you've done in getting here.

WHEN: _____ AM/PM

HOW: _____

WHERE: _____

OTHER: _____

_____

TIME: [ ]

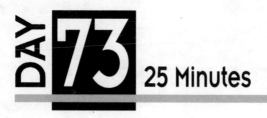

Now that you're a serious walker, you're probably noticing how many other walkers are out there. It's like when you buy a new car: it seems everyone on the planet has the same car, and same color. Especially when you're in a mall parking lot.

Don't be surprised. You've joined 14 million other Americans who know that walking is the ultimate fitness choice. Not only do you see walkers, you probably see people out racewalking (more on that in a few days) or carrying hand weights, walking poles, and stretch cords. Are these implements right for you? Perhaps.

Walkers using implements are usually trying to attain one or more of the following goals: to increase the intensity of their walks; to work their upper-body muscles more; or to simply add variety and make their walks more fun. The implements can do all of these, but consider all of your options first.

Hand weights are typically 1-to-5-pound dumbbells, or sand weights wrapped around the wrists. The quality of the workout depends on how vigorously you pump your arms. Raise them above your head, and expect a 50 percent or greater increase in calorie burn. Simply let them hang at your sides, and expect very little.

Walking poles are used like cross-country ski poles—the opposite hand and foot work together. You pole and push back with the right hand and left foot, while swinging the left hand and right foot forward. The vigor of the workout

WEIGHTS, POLES, AND CORDS—
WAYS TO INTENSIFY YOUR WALK

here depends on how hard you push back on the ground; a hearty poling action can give a 33 percent increase in intensity at a 3-mph walk.

Resistive cords pass through a padded waist belt and attach to your wrists. They are stretched during an exaggerated arm action while walking, also like cross-country skiing (they were developed by a skier as an off-snow training tool). Again, depending on your arm action, you can expect a 50 percent increase in the exercise intensity.

Finally, carrying a pack can intensify your walk. But research shows that you must carry 30 percent of your body weight in a pack to get just an 18 percent increase in calorie consumption. For a 120-pound person, that's a hefty 36-pound bag (or child). And you miss out on working the arm and shoulder muscles.

More on the implements tomorrow. For now, head out for your 25-minute walk, and enjoy how free and unencumbered you are.

WHEN: _____ AM/PM

HOW: _____

WHERE: _____

OTHER: _____

_____

TIME: ☐

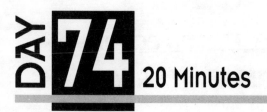

DAY 74

20 Minutes

In general, the weights, poles, and resistive cords discussed yesterday do exercise the muscles of your upper body. However, they are not miracle cures that will suddenly cause you to shed pounds or gain strength without additional effort. To get an increased calorie burn or a more intense workout, you are going to have to work harder.

Keep in mind that the research on all of the implements compares walking with them and without them at the same speed, so the increased intensity depends on *not* slowing down. The problem is, putting resistance in your hands can make your arms swing more slowly (which means slower steps, and slower walking). And if you do slow down, you may lose the increased intensity that was your goal.

The effectiveness of the exercise depends largely on how vigorously you use the implements. One study of hand weight users had them walk with identical arm movements, both with and without the weights. They found that simply moving the arms alone, without weights, created 50 to 70 percent of the increase in intensity. Adding the weights provided the rest of the increase.

You should also note two areas of concern. There are small but real increases in blood pressure when using hand weights (probably due to the gripping action of the hand and arm muscles), so if you have a history of heart disease or hypertension, don't use any of these implements without talking to your doctor first. And some physicians worry about injuries to upper-body connective tissue, especially

WHAT YOU GET OUT DEPENDS ON WHAT YOU PUT IN

in the case of heavier hand weights. The key there is to begin with very light weights (or low-resistance cords) and build up gradually.

The bottom line is that speeding up alone, and especially speeding up and bending your arms, may be the simplest way to increase the intensity of your walk. But if you feel you can't go faster (maybe your legs simply won't move any quicker, or you have physical limitations such as an old knee or hip injury), then implements are reasonable options. Just try not to slow down, and begin using them very gradually to avoid problems or upper-body injuries. And if you try them just because they're fun and it will help get you out the door, that's fine.

Speaking of which, get out for a 20-minute walk right now and log the details!

WHEN: _____ AM/PM

HOW: _____

WHERE: _____

OTHER: _____

_____

TIME: [ ]

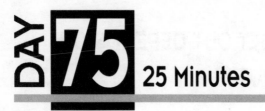

DAY 75 25 Minutes

Remember when you were a kid and Mom said, "No swimming within one hour after eating"? In fact, some people used to think any vigorous activity was inappropriate within an hour or so after eating. Perhaps this is true for certain food. A full turkey dinner, for example, might give some real discomfort before a marathon, as it jostled around in your stomach. But a small portion of high-carbohydrate food might actually be a good idea. Endurance athletes, in fact, depend on it to get through their events.

One reason that a snack might be good before you take a walk is that you may not be comfortable operating on an empty stomach. We know one college runner who was regularly getting a side stitch at her 4:00 P.M. team practices. It turned out she wasn't eating anything between her breakfast, first thing in the morning, and practice. She had classes straight through, and a laboratory session that kept her for hours. So she was starting practice on an absolutely empty stomach. It's possible that she was getting a gas bubble in her stomach, because her body thought it was time to eat and began secreting digestive juices. So she started eating a bagel right before practice, and the stitch disappeared. Her stomach had something to work on, and the bagel provided a little energy for her as well.

We're not suggesting this for everyone. But if you have problems such as a side stitch or stomach distress during your walk, or even if you are feeling hunger or a lack of

PRE-WALK SNACK—NOT NECESSARILY TABOO

energy before your scheduled walking time, don't just stick with the old one-hour rule. You may not be eating close enough to your walk, or you could be eating too close. Maybe you need a two-hour rule. Whatever the case, experiment and find out what's right for you. Of course, you need to focus on what you're eating, but more on that tomorrow.

Have a bite to eat (or not), and head out for your 25-minute walk today.

WHEN: AM/PM

HOW:

WHERE:

OTHER:

TIME:

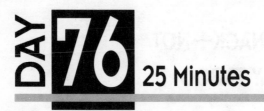

DAY 76

25 Minutes

If you do decide to try a pre-walk snack, use good judgment. Less is generally better than more, and stick with easily digestible foods such as complex carbohydrates.

Fruit is a great option. It depends on your system, but bananas seem to be a fairly universal pre-exercise favorite. Oranges are another common choice, if they're not too acidic for you. Toast or a bagel and jam is a great pre-walk meal in the morning. Even something as simple as a few crackers and peanut butter give a sense of real satisfaction. Many folks find that meat and dairy products aren't ideal before exercise because such foods take longer to digest. The point is that you will have to experiment to decide what your body prefers and tolerates best.

The other option is to have a beverage. Fruit juices are nice, but you may find you don't tolerate acidic drinks (orange and grapefruit juice) well. Also, try to stick with brands that don't have too much added sugar. A very sugary drink can actually end up sitting in your stomach, waiting to be diluted before it can pass on and be absorbed.

By the way, ingesting processed sugar such as candy and pastries right before exercise can actually cause a sudden rise in your blood sugar level. This is followed by a quick drop, however, and you can end up feeling a real "crash" (because your body has been duped into thinking it should stop supplying muscle fuel to the bloodstream). So, skip the pre-walk candy bar.

WHAT IS A SMART PRE-WALK SNACK?

There are specific beverages that are designed for before and during exercise. They're good if they have complex carbohydrates, which are better handled by your system, and if you find them to be palatable. And of course, water is a great option, because it is exactly what you need. Simply try to determine what is best for you.

Enjoy a healthy snack, and head out for your 25-minute walk.

WHEN: AM/PM

HOW:

WHERE:

OTHER:

TIME: ☐

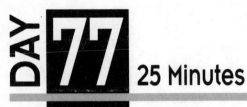

DAY 77

25 Minutes

Perhaps you've decided that your goal is to eventually walk faster than the brisk, purposeful pace in which your breathing is noticeable, but controlled. For example, if you are interested in weight loss, but can't increase the frequency and time of your walks, you may decide to pick up the pace to kick up the calorie burn. Perhaps you want the muscle-toning effects of more vigorous walking, or you simply want to cover greater distances on your walks.

The problem is, you can't just suddenly start walking faster, even though you understand the proper technique. You know to quicken your steps, push off with your toes, and maybe bend your arms. But your legs just aren't ready to turn over that much faster, and your cardiovascular system isn't ready to process all that oxygen. At least not for a full 25 minutes.

The trick is to train your body to speed up in very small increments. You probably could speed up for 30 seconds or a minute. Then you would have to slow back down to your normal walking speed for a while to catch your breath. Then you could probably speed up again for a short distance, but you'd need another rest. In fact, this is exactly the method used by competitive athletes to train to go faster.

These short bursts of faster speed are often called *intervals*. The idea is to speed up for a long enough time to get yourself breathing hard, but a short enough time that you can handle it. When you do several intervals in a row, with

HOW DO I PICK UP SPEED?

rest periods in between, this begins to stress your cardio-vascular and muscular systems and force an adaptation. The bursts can start being as short as 30 seconds, but can build up to several minutes.

One simple version of an interval workout you can do on a track is called straights and turns. You take an easy 5-to-10-minute warm-up and then pick up the tempo on the straights and ease up and walk very comfortably on the turns. Start with two or three laps' worth of this (four or six fast straightaways). If you can't walk on a track, you could use telephone poles; pick up the pace from one telephone pole to the next, then walk easily for two or three to recover.

Take a 25-minute walk, and pick up the tempo if you feel like it for a few intervals. But remember, if you're going to walk faster, an easy warm-up is essential to prepare your system for the harder efforts.

WHEN: AM/PM

HOW:

WHERE:

OTHER:

TIME:

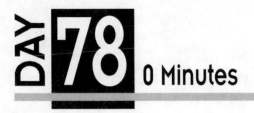

DAY 78

0 Minutes

As you become a more fit and effective walking machine, you may want to enhance your upper-body strength a bit, especially if your arms are getting more involved. There is a great deal of research indicating that even a modest strength training routine can help to reverse the loss of strength, muscle mass, and bone density that comes with inactivity and advancing age.

The wall press, a very simple exercise much like a standing push-up, might be a first step in some modest upper-body training. Rather than weights, you use your own body as the resistance against which you work. Note that your other warm-up and stretching exercises also use the body as its own resistance, so they have some strengthening effect as well.

Face a wall with your feet at shoulder width and your body at arm's length from the wall. Place your hands on the wall at shoulder height, shoulder width apart. Tighten your stomach and back muscles so you can hold your body rigid like a board, and bend your arms as you lean into the wall. Lean from the ankles so that your body remains straight, with no bend at the waist. If you can, practically touch your forehead to the wall, then press back out with your arms until they are straight. Initially try to do five presses in a row; after a short break, do another set of five. Over time you should be able to build up until you can do three sets of 10 or 15 presses.

This exercise is somewhat adjustable. To make it easier,

FOR UPPER-BODY STRENGTH, TRY WALL PRESSES

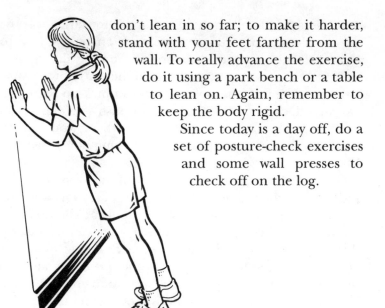

don't lean in so far; to make it harder, stand with your feet farther from the wall. To really advance the exercise, do it using a park bench or a table to lean on. Again, remember to keep the body rigid.

Since today is a day off, do a set of posture-check exercises and some wall presses to check off on the log.

WHEN: _____ AM/PM

HOW: _____

WHERE: _____

OTHER: _____

_____

DAY 79

30 Minutes

Don't let anyone tell you that walking is for fat people, or old people, or injured ex-runners, or anyone willing to accept a less than strenuous workout. You are already seeing what a great exercise walking can be, and how intense you can make it if you want to. You can pick up the pace, walk uphill, carry a pack or a child, or push a stroller. If you want to emphasize the upper-body workout, you can try hand weights, or resistive cords, or walking poles (see Day 73).

However, if you really want to crank up your workout, and remove the walking speed limit too, try racewalking. While a very vigorous, normal walk can bring you up to 4.5 or maybe 5 miles per hour, the first stage of racewalking (bending your arms) can help you reach 6 miles per hour (a 10-minute mile). Incorporating the speedy leg and hip action of the racewalk gait can allow you to go even faster. National-caliber athletes regularly move 8.5 miles per hour (7 minutes per mile) and faster, depending on the race distance.

There are two rules to competitive racewalking: one foot must always be in touch with the ground, and your supporting leg must momentarily straighten at the knee as it passes under your body. The first rule captures the visually obvious difference between a walk and a run. The second assures that a walker can't use any of the springy knee bend a runner gets on every step. With these limitations, you build your speed in racewalking by taking very

RACEWALKING—THE ATTENTION-GETTER

quick steps (sound familiar?), an even more aggressive push-off of the toes (this helps a little with stride length), and a slight front-to-back rotation of the hips. The hip rotation helps augment stride length by rotating the leg forward, and means your feet land practically one in front of the other. The arm action is a high-speed version of the hip-to-sternum arc traced by the hand, as the elbows stay bent at 90 degrees.

A simple trick to pick up the straight leg action is to stand in front of a mirror, and place all your weight on one leg with the knee straight, while leaving the other slightly bent. Then shift all your weight onto the other leg, and bend the first knee. Shift your weight back and forth quickly, barely lifting the heel of the bent knee side, and you're racewalking in place. The hip movement, by the way, should not be the side-to-side sashay made famous by so many caricatures of racewalkers.

Take a solid 30-minute walk and have some extra water afterward!

WHEN: _____ AM/PM

HOW: _____

WHERE: _____

OTHER: _____

_____

TIME: □

DAY 80 25 Minutes

Over the next several days we'll do a quick review of the key habits you've been working to form over the 90 days of this program. We'll call them the Cardinal Rules, although they really aren't rules. One thing about fitness walking as an exercise is that it is ultimately flexible, allowing it to fit your needs and lifestyle. However, these rules will be useful guidelines as you continue to walk after you're done with the book. The first of these guidelines is that you should walk as often as you can, and be more active in general.

To fully benefit from walking you have to make it a part of your daily life, and that means not thinking about *whether* you'll take a walk that day, but *when*. And because walking is so physically forgiving, six days a week is a reasonable goal and a healthy goal. You also know to look for every opportunity in life to be more active, and to be especially conscious of day-to-day activity.

As part of the plan not to skip walks, you've learned to use a training log. Whether you've just checked off when you do your workout, or recorded every detail from the beginning warm-up move to the last stretch, a log is an honest assessor of your efforts. Its purpose is to help you maintain your six-day-per-week schedule. Start thinking

CARDINAL RULE NO. 1—DON'T SKIP DAYS, AND BE MORE ACTIVE

now of how you will make up your own training log when you're done with our 90 days. More ideas on this later. For now, take a 25-minute walk, warm up before and stretch after as you please, and think about what you'd put in your own custom training log.

WHEN: AM/PM

HOW:

WHERE:

OTHER:

TIME:

DAY 81

30 Minutes

The basis of your walking is a healthy technique, and the basis of that technique is good posture. Of all the exercises you've learned, the posture check may be the most important, because that will help you maintain a healthy body alignment all the time, not just while you're walking. Remember the basics:

—Hold your shoulders low and relaxed, but don't slouch.

—Do not lean forward from the hips.

—Keep your eyes forward, not down.

—Tighten those abdominal muscles to flatten your lower back, and no shelf-butt.

Remember, all the things just listed are natural elements of how your body is designed to walk. The problem is that we create so many bad postural habits—slumping in chairs, hunching over keyboards, slouching as we stand in line, with our too-heavy bellies arching our backs—that we're simply relearning the basics as we work on good walking posture.

As you speed up your walks, keep that healthy posture, even with a more advanced technique. Keep a natural-length stride, let your speed come from quicker steps, think of pushing off the back foot, and let your arms bend at the elbow to shorten the arm pendulums and quicken your steps even more.

If you want to know what other exercises to explore beyond the ones we've shown you, the first to consider are

CARDINAL RULE NO. 2—SPEED COMES FROM TECHNIQUE; TECHNIQUE IS BUILT ON POSTURE

more advanced abdominal exercises. The days of 100 ballistic sit-ups are long gone, but if you have a few more minutes to add to your daily routine, some simple abdominal crunches would be a perfect supplement to the posture-check exercise you've learned.

Do a few posture checks, then head out and walk for 30 minutes.

WHEN: _____ AM/PM

HOW: _____

WHERE: _____

OTHER: _____

_____

TIME:

The best way to reach and maintain a healthy weight is to combine a healthy, moderate diet with regular daily exercise. Drinking a lot of water is helpful to both of those; it's a key element to the diet, and pivotal raw material for an exercising body, as you are learning through your program.

Though the changes in your weight and health won't come overnight, this rule will produce changes that last a lifetime. Remember that a healthy diet just means back to the basics. Break the fat and sugar habit. Instead:

—Focus on lots of fruits and vegetables—a great way to get your complex carbohydrates.

—Search out whole grains and legumes.

—Let water fill the void when you are thirsty and not hungry, and any other time you think of drinking it.

Have patience that the diet and exercise are working now, and will continue to work. In fact, this is the pivotal time in your program, because your exercise bouts are getting long enough to really impact your fitness, especially if you are thinking about your breathing and cranking up the intensity two or three days a week. Now that you're walking 30 minutes, you're burning a significant number of calories during your exercise, but you're also building the muscle, which is a great calorie-burning tissue even when you're not exercising.

In a sense, you've now paid the dues and gotten in good enough shape to *really* get in shape. So reap the benefits,

CARDINAL RULE NO. 3—COMBINE EXERCISE WITH A HEALTHY DIET AND LOTS OF WATER

and enjoy the accelerating effects of healthy diet and exercise. Today, go burn some of that healthy diet that you're eating and sweat out some of the water you've been drinking with a nice 25-minute walk!

WHEN: _____ AM/PM

HOW: _____

WHERE: _____

OTHER: _____

_____

TIME: ☐

DAY 83 — 30 Minutes

Vary the venue, and vary the workout. These two tips are the best ways to keep your walking routine interesting and enjoyable, both mentally and physically.

Seek out new places to walk, look for great weekend walking adventures, such as parks or conservation lands, or go so far as to plan a vacation around walking—inn to inn through New England, for example, or a hiking exploration of Yellowstone National Park.

Seeking out new people to walk with also affects your walking venue. This can be as elaborate as joining a walking club, or as simple as getting involved with a bunch of regular walkers in your neighborhood every morning. Whatever you choose, always be on the lookout for ways to keep your walking environment stimulating and exciting.

Varying the workout is a great way to keep your walks physically stimulating, because you are constantly giving your body variety. Remember the hard/easy principle. Even if you only vary the intensity of your walks, faster some days and easier on others, it's one step in keeping your body fresh and active from day to day. But remember F.I.T.—you can vary **F**requency, **I**ntensity, and **T**ime in myriad ways. Walk for longer amounts of time some days, shorter amounts on others, to avoid feeling stale. Pick hilly courses to work the quads and calves, then alternate with flatter and easier loops to give those muscles a break. Walk an interval workout at the local track with friends on Saturday mornings, or simply do your 30-minute walk there. The

CARDINAL RULE NO. 4—KEEP IT FUN

bottom line is to mix up the physical stresses on your body, to keep it constantly adapting and getting in better shape, and to mix up the environment for your head, so you never, ever, ever get bored with walking.

Whatever you do, make walking fun! Head out for an interesting 30-minute walk right now!

WHEN: _____ AM/PM

HOW: _____

WHERE: _____

OTHER: _____

_____

TIME: [ ]

DAY 84

25 Minutes

You've learned a wide range of tools with which to build and supplement your daily walking routine. You don't have to use these tools every day, but they are there for you, and you should remember them because they may come in handy.

The tools can be another way to keep your walking healthy and fun by keeping your body in good shape for walking. They fall into three categories:

1) Warm-up exercises:
   —Ankle circles
   —Trunk rotations
   —Arm circles

Use these particularly if you're feeling tight or sore, but also think about them on a day when you're not very motivated and not sure you even want to take your walk. The mere act of starting a warm-up exercise can get your blood flowing, elevate your heart rate, begin to raise your mental awareness, and bring your motivation level up.

2) Strength exercises:
   —Posture check, a pivotal exercise that you should do as often as you think of it to help strengthen your abdominal muscles
   —Wall press, the upper-body exercise for the muscles that don't get quite as much work in the normal walking movement

CARDINAL RULE NO. 5—REMEMBER ALL THE TOOLS

3) Stretches:
   —Toe point (for the shin)
   —Calf stretch
   —Hamstring stretch
   —Thigh stretch
   —Shoulder stretch

These are important to maintain the health and range of motion of the muscles that you're using in your walking, and you should do them when you feel the need. But it would be great to get in the habit of doing them two or three times a week after your workouts. Remember, always stretch after the muscles are warm and compliant.

For today, practice whichever exercises you choose, and take a 25-minute walk.

WHEN: _____ AM/PM

HOW: _____

WHERE: _____

OTHER: _____

_____

TIME: [ ]

DAY 85 0 Minutes

Eleven weeks ago, we suggested you go to the doctor. You may have balked, for fear of getting news you didn't want to hear. But for the past eleven weeks you've been committed to a progressively more demanding program of walking. You've been thinking of healthier eating and drinking gallons of water. And you've generally been more active. If that's all true, it's going to show, especially to your doctor.

That's not to say you should expect *huge* changes. Remember that because you've been building up gradually, you only reached 30-minute walks in the last two weeks. And only you know how diligent you've been about your diet and other activities. But if you are doing all those things, expect to see a change. More important, if you simply maintain all of those habits, the next six months could produce the greatest results of all.

You've built a foundation of conditioning that will let you go out and average 30 minutes of walking every day. If you begin to accumulate weeks of regular exercise like that, especially if a couple of walks each week are vigorous, then you can really expect to see your weight drop and your stamina improve.

Look back on Day 10 and check out the numbers from that first visit to the doctor. Then make an appointment to have those same measurements and statistics taken again. Or, even better, make an appointment for three to six months from now, to *really* measure some progress.

SEEING THE DOCTOR AGAIN TO CHART RESULTS

But no resting on your laurels now. If you missed a day last week, walk today and record it. Or check off for calling the doctor to make a follow-up appointment (and for drinking some extra water).

WHEN: _____ AM/PM

HOW: _____

WHERE: _____

OTHER: _____

_____

TIME: [ ]

DAY 86 — 30 Minutes

Seven weeks ago (Day 37) I suggested you go to the track and measure your walking speed. Now, you may not be at all interested in trying to walk fast, which is absolutely great. The goal here is not to make everyone a speed walker. The pure fun of walking for many of us is that there are so many health benefits at a purposeful but comfortable pace. The talk about faster walking is for those really interested in fitness benefits—the ability to sustain a higher level of activity for a longer time, without getting winded or fatigued, or for people who absolutely feel they must calculate speed in order to feel the psychological benefits of walking.

Whether you consciously think about speeding up or not, you might be surprised to know that you're probably walking faster now than when you started, whether you've tried to or not. If you now comfortably walk 30 minutes per day, and your body has grown accustomed to this activity, your heart may be stronger, your leg muscles may be stronger and have more capillaries, there may be more blood flowing through your veins, and you may have better, healthier posture because of all the exercises you do. All of these contribute to a faster walk.

Head to the track, and walk one or two easy laps to warm up. Then wow the crowd with some ankle circles, trunk rotations, and arm circles, and any stretches you feel are necessary to really impress on-lookers (remember, it's okay to stretch once you're warmed up). Then knock off four

IF YOU WANT TO, CHECK YOUR SPEED

laps at the fastest pace you normally use during a daily walk—no faster—and time them. Finally, walk enough more laps to reach a 30-minute total.

If you compare your minute-per-mile (or mile-per-hour) pace to Day 37, remember the weather may also affect your speed. If today is hot and humid, or windy and frigid, and the other day was calm and comfortable, today's time will suffer a bit by comparison.

WHEN: _____ AM/PM

HOW: _____

WHERE: _____

OTHER: _____

_____

TIME: [ ]

DAY 87 30 Minutes

You are walking 30 minutes a day, six days a week. By now this should seem comfortable yet it is enough walking for significantly better health and well-being. This amount of walking meets the American College of Sports Medicine's quota for long-term health benefits and you can maintain the 30-minute, 6-day-per-week routine for as long as you like.

However, keep in mind Cardinal Rule #4—keep your routine fun. To vary the venue and vary the workout suggests that although 30 minutes a day does the basic job, you may want to mix your walks up just to maintain your interest and keep improving your fitness.

One approach is to work toward longer walks. You can set 30 minutes as your daily minimum, and work up to 45-minute and one-hour walks occasionally. By now you know the pattern—one week increase a few walks to 35–40 minutes, then the next week go up to 45–50 minutes. But you can leave 30-minute walks sprinkled in during the week—now that you're a walking machine, they'll seem like recovery!

Perhaps you'll get really hardcore, and decide to prepare for some weekend all-day hikes. But even if you're building up to a three- or five-hour hike, you can still plan your training weeks following the same rules: Don't increase the total time more than 10–20 percent per week (although as your weekly total grows larger, so does the amount you can safely add—three hours of walking this week means a 20–

ADDING TIME TO YOUR PROGRAM

30-minute increase next week is fine); alternate harder and easier days; throw in an easier week now and then, where you don't increase the total at all. And if you decide to prepare for an especially long walk (say, a ten-mile charity walk) you may choose to focus your weekly increases on one or two longer weekend walks, rather than spread them over the week. Using the same principles you've used to go from walking nothing to covering 30 minutes per day, you eventually can build up to walking several hours in a day. Remember Ron Cook, who walked the Boston Marathon in 4½ hours?

If you are going to take on something that vigorous, you may find it best to actually write out a plan. For today, get in your 30-minute walk, and think about your future walking goals.

WHEN: _____ AM/PM

HOW: _____

WHERE: _____

OTHER: _____

_____

TIME: ☐

DAY 88 30 Minutes

Another way to keep your fitness walking routine interesting is to add intensity to your walks. Here are some options. If you want to try increasing your walking speed, concentrating on technique and picking up the pace on your regular walks is one way to begin. Just don't forget to warm up if you're picking up the tempo. But it may be more fun to head to the track for some straights and turns, or to use the telephone-pole intervals on the road, which allow you to focus on quick steps, and bending the arms, while keeping you from getting too wiped out. If you find speed intriguing, give racewalking a try—you may be a natural. There are good books and videos available, and plenty of local and regional walking clubs full of people delighted to teach and walk with newcomers (racewalkers seem to be an evangelical lot). In fact, simply going to a local track and walking briskly may hook you up with a local club, many of which now have walkers of every ilk, from racers to hikers to mall strollers.

Maybe it's not speed, but hills that excite you. Then get out and grind up some inclines—just don't forget to stretch afterward. Think about getting out into different parts of town or the country if you like hills, to vary the venue and reward yourself with a view if you're going to burn all those calories. Even if you don't want to climb mountains, some lighter off-road hiking could do the trick.

Perhaps you really feel equipment will add variety to your walks. Then consider poles, cords, or weights, but try to

ADDING INTENSITY TO YOUR PROGRAM

borrow them from a walking friend or neighbor before you make major purchases. If you hook up with a local walking club you are bound to find someone who's willing to share.

Maybe something as routine as pushing a stroller or carrying a child on your back is the perfect intensifier for you, which is fine. The key is to find out what makes adding intensity fun and do it.

After a few posture checks take a 30-minute walk, maintaining flawless posture and perfect technique throughout.

WHEN: _____ AM/PM

HOW: _____

WHERE: _____

OTHER: _____

_____

TIME: [ ]

DAY 89 30 Minutes

Whether you decide to continue the progression of this book and make your walks longer, or to crank up the intensity on your walks, or choose to stay right here at brisk 30-minute walks is your choice. What will keep you excited about walking and interested in getting out every day is all that's important. But whether or not you increase the time or the intensity, that third variable, frequency, should not be considered a matter of choice.

Remember Cardinal Rule #1—don't skip workouts, and be more active. If you never take a step faster than 2 mph, and never walk longer than 30 minutes, make sure you keep walking six days per week. If you absolutely, positively have to miss more than one walk in a week, make up for it by always seeking every opportunity to be more active: ride your bike to the store; stack some firewood; go dancing; run up the stairs to beat the folks that took the elevator for one floor; wash your windows; get off the bus a stop early; shovel that snow (and warm up before, and gently stretch afterward—it counts!); push a kid on a swing; paddle a canoe; weed the garden.

In deciding what to continue to do with your walking, remember the subtle difference between walking for health and walking for fitness. Comfortable 30-minute walks taken regularly are a great start for "heart" health and longevity. But there is a direct correlation between the vigor of your exercise and continuing improvements in health and fitness. The more often your walks are brisk

TO STAY F.I.T., MAINTAIN A FREQUENT WALKING SCHEDULE

workouts, in which you notice your breathing and effort, and the more accumulated minutes you exercise each week, the lower the risk of heart disease and premature death. Are there guarantees? Of course not, because this is based on statistics. But you certainly know how to make the numbers work in your favor.

First and foremost, keep walking, and keep doing it regularly. Second, look for every other way you can think of to be more active. And third, if you can muster some more vigorous walks, or more total walking time in a week, it will be worth the effort you invest.

Warm up and take a brisk 30-minute walk today. Do some posture checks and wall presses afterward to make it a total workout.

WHEN: _____ AM/PM

HOW: _____

WHERE: _____

OTHER: _____

_____

TIME: ☐

DAY 90 30 Minutes

Today's the last day you'll fill in the log in this book. When you walk tomorrow, you should begin your own log. Decide what you do and don't like about keeping a log, and make one up that matches your style.

At a minimum, you should keep some record of the days you do and don't walk. That allows you to keep tabs on your six-days-per-week schedule, and notice if you're getting sloppy about missing days. Beyond that, the details are up to you. As you may have seen already, the more you record, the more useful the log can be. The basic elements we've recorded here are how long you walked, the location, and how you felt. The last one is important in keeping an eye on any budding injuries. Adding who you went with, the time of day, or other observations give more flavor to the entry.

My grandfather keeps a daily log (not a diary, just his daily activities and contacts) and he even records the weather. I did the same when training seriously, since it sometimes impacted the workout (I allowed for slower times on really hot days, for example). We both found that simple additions added great color to our entries, making recollections of specific events more vivid. You may find other seemingly mundane observations will do the same for you.

You can put your log on a 12-month calendar if you tend toward leaner entries. Notes like "W-35" and "Yrd-1 hr." for a 35-minute walk and one hour of yard work will easily

CREATE YOUR OWN TRAINING LOG

fit in the corner of the date boxes. On the other hand, if you are going to record full details you may want to use a small notebook or three-ring binder. Any stationery store will have weekly calendars that are small and convenient, and athletic footwear stores often carry specifically designed runner's and walker's log books. There are also computer programs designed to be used as daily logs (they will even chart your progress and tally totals), or you could create your own on a spreadsheet.

Finally, make sure to create a routine, so that your log fills the same role this book has for you. Whether you fill it in right after your walk, or every night before lights out, make it a habit that you never miss. Then you will be encouraged never to miss your walk, either.

Enjoy a 30-minute walk today and record whatever makes your heart content in the log.

WHEN: _____ AM/PM

HOW: _____

WHERE: _____

OTHER: _____

_____

TIME: [ ]

30 Minutes

Now it's up to you. There will be no book peering over your shoulder, reminding you to walk every day, but chances are you won't need one. Because if you have done all of the walks recommended so far, you are now truly a walker.

That does not mean you are some fanatic whom people don't want to talk to at parties because the only thing he or she talks about is walking (and how many calories there are in the dip). You simply have found the healthful benefits and rejuvenated spirit that regular, daily activity brings to your life.

You should feel great pride at what you've accomplished in the last three months. Take a moment to savor that accomplishment. You have gone from no walking at all, to comfortably cruising through 30 minutes a day or more. Walk today, and you will have done it for six straight days— exactly your goal when you set out. That's a testimony to your discipline, perseverance, and desire to do something positive for your health and well-being.

What you do with your future fitness walking program is entirely up to you. But you can be sure that you know how to do it safely and intelligently.

Write to us and tell us about how you have made walking work in your life and what it has done for you. Reach us at:

90-Day Fitness Walking Program
Walking Magazine
9–11 Harcourt Street
Boston MA 02116

CONGRATULATIONS—YOU ARE AN ACCOMPLISHED FITNESS WALKER!

Finally, be proud enough of what you have done to share it with others. Just as you may have been hesistant before you started on this program, you probably have friends or colleagues that are also apprehensive about exercise. Yet you are a living example of how easy and attainable a healthier lifestyle can be. So invite a friend on a walk, and share with them how great this exercise is! Happy walking.

RESOURCES

For information about trails and facilities in national parks, write:

National Park Service
Office of Inquiries
P.O. Box 37127
Washington DC 20013-7127

The American Volksport Association hosts many noncompetitive 10-kilometer (6.2-mile) walks throughout the year, around the country. There are many active regional clubs, and new members of any experience, fitness, and interest level are welcome. For information write them at:

American Volksport Association
1001 Pat Booker Road, Suite 101
Universal City TX 78148
(800) 830-WALK

Information on racewalking clubs around the U.S., events, and educational resources such as tapes and videos are available from:

North American Race Walk Foundation
P.O. Box 50312
Pasadena CA 91115-0312

For ultra-distance walking, consider training for the Viere Daagse (4-days) march. It's a 40-kilometer-per-day, 4-day non-competitive event held each July in Nijmegen, Holland, with over 35,000 people participating! (The 80th annual event will be in 1996.)

This is the premier event in a series of multi-day marches, which also occur in Belgium, Switzerland, Luxemburg, England, Denmark, Ireland, Austria, Norway, and Japan. The International Marching League oversees all of these, and can be contacted at the following address.

International Marching League (I.M.L.)
Postbus 61533
2506 AM Den Haag
The Netherlands
Tel. 070-360 4141 Fax. 070-356 2754

Walking Magazine is the only magazine in the U.S. written specifically for walkers.

Walking Magazine
9–11 Harcourt Street
Boston, MA 02116
Subscriptions: (800) 678-0881